Brain Candy

BRAIN CANDY

A Memoir

By Deirdre Allen Timmons

Lemonbird Press

Printed in the United States of America
First Printing, 2019

Cover Design: Annette Kraus
Interior Design: Abigail Carter

ISBN: 978-0-9911050-5-2
1. Cancer 2. Self Help 3. Dementia 4. Humor

Lemonbird Press
Seattle, WA 98178

for Rose

❦ TABLE OF CONTENTS ❦

CHAPTER 1

Spin doctors

"Hi, I know we just met, but I have an awkward question," I say into the phone.

"Shoot," says the voice on the other end.

"How did I get home last night?"

"You walked home," he responds. "Actually, I walked you home."

"OK, Awkward Question Number Two," I continue. "Did you come into my apartment?"

"Noooo, why?" he asks.

"OK, bear with me," I say. "Is there any chance I was roofied last night and something else happened? Like, maybe I went back out after you dropped me off?"

"I don't think so," he assures me. "We watched the waitress cork the wine and I certainly didn't roofy you!"

"So as far as you know, nobody came into my Airbnb with me?" I press on.

"I just dropped you off. I don't know what you did after that. You seemed pretty out of it, so I assume you went to bed," he reasons. "Why? What's up?"

I'm in LA in pre-pre-production for my next film. I'm a fish out of water here: Middle-aged, pale, not petite, prone to acne, kind of a doofus tripping over my own feet and constantly cracking childish jokes.

I am clearly not a local when I stroll Hollywood and Vine.

But I'm a filmmaker, and eventually projects compel me to come to the City of Angels so I can duke it out with the devils. Making the circuit of dinners, parties and meetings, I'm now in the early stages of figuring out my fund-raising strategy, brainstorming with friends, talking to anyone who will listen, plotting potential cast and crew. Sometimes I know the people I'm meeting, sometimes I don't.

Last night, I dined with a producer. Nice guy. Genuine. Funny. Creative. Cool. Just good peeps. So I am confuzzled, to say the least, when I wake up the morning after our dinner nauseous, confused, exhausted, dizzy, and covered in bruises. There are no signs of struggle in the small Airbnb I've rented that's filled with brightly painted furniture and simple art, which evokes a whiff of Southern France meets Cabo San Lucas in Venice Beach.

"Sorry to belabor this questioning," I continue, "but I woke up this morning covered in bruises. I believe someone may have beaten me up last night, maybe after you dropped me off?"

"What?" he asks.

"Yeah, it's the weirdest thing. I look like a junkie on the street … I have dark circles under my eyes and bruises all over my body."

"Hmmm," he considers. "Has this ever happened before?"

"No."

"Do you want me to take you to a hospital, maybe just to get checked out?" he offers.

"No, but thanks," I say, now sitting on the toilet to check my panties for any sign of further violation. They are clean clean clean. "Did we drink a lot?"

I only remember drinking a couple of glasses of wine. But see that's the problem with alcohol — drink too much and you only remember those first couple of drinks and the rest becomes a montage of vague scenes.

"We shared one bottle of a nice cab at an outdoor café in Santa Monica with a cheese plate and some delightful conversation, then we walked back," he says with an edge of kindness in his voice. "I highly doubt anybody beat you up last night. When I left you, you looked ready for the sack."

Though I've only recently met this man, I trust him. I turn my back to the mirror while holding my phone, craning my neck to study my black-and-blue arms.

"OK. Well, I head back to Seattle today so I'll just — I don't know — think about it, maybe go to my doctor there," I fib. I hate going to the doctor and I only do it if I think I'm dying, which to date has been never.

Secretly, I'm thinking I can't handle my booze anymore and last night I must have just fallen (into a thresher?) once I got back to my place.

"It was lovely meeting you. Thank you so much for putting up with my neurotic questioning," I say, "and maybe next time I'm in town we can have coffee."

"Sounds great," he says. "Definitely go to a doctor. Nice meeting you too. Good luck and let me know how your project progresses."

"Will do. Take care, " I say before pushing the End Call on my phone.

I board my plane back to Seattle and study my arms. I should've worn a long-sleeved shirt. The passenger next to me eyeballs my arms and immediately dives into the in-flight magazine.

"Would you like a drink?" the flight attendant asks.

"White wine?" I sheepishly ask, thinking, *See, Deirdre, this is why you're always dizzy. Too. Much. Booze.*

Upon arriving in Seattle, I trip trying to get my luggage off the conveyer belt.

"Can I help you?" asks a man watching me struggle.

"Oh yes. Thank you," I respond, relieved for the help.

I weave my way to arrivals and wait for my ride.

"Welcome back to Sunny Seattle!" jokes my husband, Jack, as he steps out of his car at the Sea-Tac arrivals platform on a rainy May afternoon and pops open the trunk. I can barely lift my bag.

"Can you get it?" I ask, opening the passenger door.

He gives me a quick kiss and throws my suitcase in the trunk.

Jack and I met more than 25 years ago in a nightclub. I was 21. He was 27. For me, it was love at first sight. He was tall, handsome, charismatic, speaking in a soft Southern drawl *and* he offered to buy me a drink (which doesn't happen often in the Seattle bar scene). We danced and went to a local Italian restaurant for pastries and coffee. When I got home at 3 a.m. that morning, I woke up my parents.

"Get up! Get up! Get up!" I demanded, pulling my parents out of bed. "I'm getting married!"

"You're drunk," my father flatly stated, trying to shoo me away.

"I know," I responded, dragging both parents downstairs and opening a bottle of champagne. "But that doesn't change a thing! I'm still getting married! I'm in love! I'm going to have children! You're going to be grandparents again! Cheers!!!!"

While my parents didn't believe me that night, they laughed along with my exuberance and toasted my dubious marriage to this stranger whose name I couldn't quite remember. "Jack? John? Jim? Jerry? Something with a J," I told them. "I'm in love with Jacknmrrry!" I sang, tossing back my bubbly and dancing circles around my parents.

One year later, I made good on that random declaration as I walked down the aisle in the small chapel at my high school alma mater, an all-girls boarding school, and joined that same man (Jack, it turns out) at the altar. After 25 years, 15 moves, several academic degrees, and one daughter who has already sprouted like a sunflower, dwarfing me in her 6-foot shadow, Jack and I are still each other's biggest cheerleaders in life.

"Whoa, look at you," Jack says as we leave the airport. I'm now 47 and he's 53. "You look like shit. Do you feel OK?"

"Tell me about it. I feel worse than I look," I tell him.

"Hungover?" he presumes.

"Prolly," I admit, turning on the seat warmer and rolling down the window of his large green Mercedes because I'm inexplicably cold and hot at the same time.

"How'd it go?" he asks. I know he's hoping to hear I secured a producer or some financing or just anything promising for my next film, a musical narrative about male burlesque dancers.

This will be my third film. My first movie was a lighthearted musical documentary about ten women learning burlesque called "A Wink and a Smile." I never released my second documentary about female comediennes in LA because, well, because I didn't like it even though I mortgaged my house and spent two years on it. Now, hoping to redeem myself in the world of film, I am returning to burlesque — but this time I'm planning an eye-popping musical about the men who take the stage and take it off.

Lest you think I was always a paparazzi-shunning filmmaker married to my first love and traveling the globe in search of glittery dreams, you would be wrong. I've done hard time mucking around in pursuit of a gritty story. After graduating college and floundering for a few years, I launched a high-profile career in newspapers covering wedding announcements, obits, police blotters, and eventually actual news about such heady topics as sewer district shenanigans and the local library's storytime hours. Once I even covered a shooting!

In the early '90s when this mysterious, nay, this suspicious force called the World Wide Web was sneaking into nerdy home computers fed by some mysterious uber-computer overlord that channeled endless information (given a phone line and a lot of time), I transitioned into being an Internet reporter. Saying my goodbyes in the newsroom, my peers looked at me with heartfelt pity trying to warn me, "Deirdre, I've heard about this thing called the 'Information SuperHighway.' It's going nowhere. Once you leave newspapers, you'll never get back in."

Well, they were right about that. I never returned to the old ink-stained profession, and Internet reporting turned into magazine writing, which eventually led me to screenwriting, where I could indulge my zest for big stories, funny stories, touching stories, but most importantly, stories that would make you tap your toes and walk away with a song in your heart.

Meanwhile, my daughter Rosemary came into our world, and Jack and I began the challenging road of trying to 'have it all.' After almost three years of raising a baby and working at Microsoft editing a restaurant section for a website called Sidewalk, we decided I should stay home. I would tend to the domestic duties of nurturing our practically perfect baby. Jack would play the role of 'Mule Boy,' bringing home the ducats to put gruel on the table and rags on our backs.

Rose was very patient with us. Child Protective Services probably should have been alerted to the sketchy menu I provided (Hello Kraft Macaroni and Cheese!) and our growing fascination with post-bedtime martinis. But somehow, we muddled through with a lot of laughs and love. Rose grew (and grew and grew), she sailed through high school, I chased my little dreams behind a camera … and Jack wisened up.

Everybody was having more fun than he was.

"I wanna chase a dream too," he shared one night.

"OK, doing …..?" I asked, thinking, *Here it is! The Midlife Crisis! What'll it be? An open marriage? A Tesla? Maybe a move to Cabo?* He'd never talked about pursuing this thing called "a dream." I was the artist chasing rainbow unicorns. He was the engineer looking at ones and zeroes. I made life fun. He paid for it. He had never talked about having a dream.

"I want to smoke," he said.

"Honey, you do smoke," I answered, nodding at the cigar in his hand.

"No. I want to smoke meat." As a native Texan, he explained, he missed the slow-smoked barbecue of his youth.

So he bought a smoker that would smoke enough meat for 20 people. We had lots of parties, and the minute the meat came out of the smoker, it was consumed by our hungry guests as quickly as he could slice it.

Then he bought a bigger smoker — this one would smoke enough brisket for 40 people.

As his obsession to smoke grew, so did the smokers in our back-yard. He purchased a used offset smoker from a local restaurant that was no longer smoking meats. Dubbed "Big Bertha," she could smoke enough ribs, chicken, brisket and pork for 200 people. To accommodate his growing interest, Jack created The Seattle Bris-ket Experience, hosting barbecue raves at local breweries and event spaces. He'd hire bands and sell tickets, and the rise he got out of his newfound 'hobby' (not to mention his followers) began to demand all of his attention, clouding his focus on doing what he had done for 30 years — work in high-tech.

On the way home from the airport, he suppresses his excitement to tell me about another smoker he found online. This one could smoke enough meat for — I shit you not — 1,000 people. He'd been texting me during my whole trip to get a read on my approval-meter for what was becoming a very expensive hobby.

"You didn't answer my question. How was LA?" he asks, rolling up my window as the rain pours into the car.

"You know LA. They hate my work. Mention something gay or musical and their eyes roll back in their heads and they start fixating on the nearest exit," I lament. "Hey, check out my bruises."

"Oh my god!" he exclaims. "What happened?"

"Right? I dunno. I had a nice calm dinner, went back to the apartment early, and woke up with these bruises," I explain.

"That's just weird," he says. "I mean, really, what happened?"

"Nothing," I say. "I think I'm just drinking too much, it's thinning my blood and it's causing bruising. You know, like my mom's meds cause her to bruise. I haven't been beaten up … I just gotta quit drinking."

"Or hang out with nicer people," he jokes.

As soon as we get home I hop in my own car to visit my mom. My mother, Kathy, still lives in the '70s faux Tudor home that I grew up in on Mercer Island — one floating bridge away from Seattle. She has advanced Alzheimer's and can never be left alone — her every need requires assistance (though she still insists on doing her own makeup). She has five caregivers: myself; my nieces Laura and Kimmie; Kimmie's husband Dennis; and a homecare worker. While I manage her team of caregivers, I also spend a few days a week bathing her, doing her shopping, laundering her clothes, organizing her house, walking her dog, paying her bills, but most importantly, trying to shift her mood, which is often gloomy.

"Hi Mom, how is my favorite person in the whole wide world?" I ask, hugging her.

"Where you been, Rin Tin Tin?" she asks. "I've been waiting for you. Listen, I wanna go home."

"You are home, Mom," I tell her. "You've lived here for 40 years."

"God dammit! Quit saying that," she bursts, on the brink of tears. "Take me to MY home.

"What does 'your' home look like?" I ask her.

"Oh you know! It's yellow," she says. "It's just down the street from here."

Sometimes, I agree to take mom home. I make her potty. I put on her coat. I put her in the car. And I start driving.

"Mind if we go to Starbucks on the way?" I ask. "I want a chai tea, and I'll bet you wouldn't turn down a mocha latte."

"Yay!" she cheers. She loves Starbucks.

So we sit by the fire and sip our drinks and tell tall tales, and when we finish, we go home.

By the time we arrive at her real-in-life-but-not-real-to-Kathy's home, she's tuckered out and has completely forgotten about wanting to go to some other home, possibly her childhood home.

As the urgency to "go home" intensifies, I've learned to shorten the trick and just take her to the bathroom. That short errand resets her mental looping, and she forgets she has to get home. Or I walk her to the mailbox, pick up the mail, and walk her back home. Or I just put her coat on and take it back off.

As she catches on to my tricks, she develops a few tricks of her own. She's started getting up in the middle of the night and whispering to her dog Arthur, "Come on Arthur, let's go home." Tiptoeing down the stairs, Kimmie (my niece) or Dennis (her husband) have to jump up and guide her back to bed — much to her irritation.

Neighbors are on full alert to walk Kathy home if she is found wandering. The police are familiar with our calls of the grandma escapee. We even put locks on the inside of doors and windows so she can't sneak out, but she's good ... she's figured out how to escape when we get sloppy and don't have the house in full lockdown while showering or having a private moment in the loo.

"Oh boy, am I dizzy. Everything's going woo-woo-woo," she says.

"Yes, you've been telling me you're dizzy for quite some time."

"No, D-D, this just started," she argues, calling me by my child-hood nickname.

"Nope you dope, Mom. You've been dizzy for a few years now," I assure her.

When my mother was in her late 40s, she got a little queer — blowing up over a lost shoe that was right in front of her face, getting lost driving home from Roberto's Pizza where we'd been dining for years, and most horrifyingly, forgetting our birthdays, graduations and the occasional Christmas. With a healthy streak of Alzheimer's running thick in the veins of my maternal family, my brother Sam and I would whisper conspiratorially, "Alzheimer's," when she couldn't remember how to use her cash card or how to gas up the car, or even how to open an umbrella.

We just thought we were being bratty little insult meisters behind our mother's back, but it turns out, we were right. Though it took the medical community another 20 years to acknowledge what my brother and I had identified in the 1980s, my mom actually did have Alzheimer's. Now she is far down the very frustrating path of losing her mind.

"Then why don't they do something about my dizziness?" she asks, repeating her litany of standard questions.

"Well, problem is, it's a symptom of your disease, and there's really nothing the doctors can do for it."

"What disease?" she asks.

"Alzheimer's," I tell her honestly. This is a conversation we have many times a day. And though Mom was a top-notch nurse all of her adult life, she no longer has any recall of her medical knowledge. "It's a brain disease that you've had for years."

"Oh, have I?" she asks.

"Yup," I tell her.

"Well, that's the shits," she says. "And it makes me dizzy?"

"Yup. But if it makes you feel any better, I'm dizzy too."

"Why are you dizzy?"

"Dunno," I confess. "Maybe I have early Alzheimer's like you did."

"Oh no, that's terrible," she twists her face. "But you look great! You're so skinny."

"Why thank you! I've lost almost 30 pounds."

Kathy has had me on diets since I was a child, and for her, how thin I am is a measure of how beautiful I am — and at times how successful I am.

"How did you lose the weight?" she asks, clearly impressed.

"Funny thing, I went on a diet a little over a month ago and the weight just fell off," I tell her. "I haven't even really tried. I'm just not hungry."

"Well, whatever you're doing, it looks fabulous," she croons. Even though Kathy has lost complete track of where she is — or even who she is — Alzheimer's has not been able to uproot my mother's vanity. Quite shockingly, Kathy still marks her weight on a calendar by her bed every night. "Keep doing it, kid! Ya look good skinny. By the way, where's Fred?"

Fred is my father, who died the previous autumn. My mother asks where he is probably 100 times a day, and I tell her the truth — most of the time. "Dad died in October, Mom."

"He did?" she asks, as I shake my head in confirmation. "Shit-house mouse. Did I know that?"

"Yes," I tell her. "But if you want, I'll quit telling you he's passed on, because every time I tell you it makes you sad. Mom, do you want me to tell you he's still alive?"

"No," she says, tearing up. "Don't do that, D-D. Tell me the truth. What did he die of?"

"Diabetes, Mom," I tell her. "Because he didn't listen to you and he didn't eat right and he didn't exercise. Because of that he became very unhealthy, then very ill, then he died. He was 77."

"Was there a funeral?" she asks, becoming increasingly agitated and mournful.

"Yes, and you went," I tell her, scrolling through the photos on my iPhone. "See, here's a picture of you at his funeral. That's Sam, your son. And that's me, your daughter."

"I'll be damned. He was 77?" she asks, trying to piece this story together before she loses track of the conversation.

"Yes," I answer, distilling the story for her, once again. "Your husband Fred died peacefully in his sleep at 77."

"How old am I?" She wipes her cheeks dry, distracted by her new question.

"You're 77, Mom," I tell her.

"Hell's bells! Am I really?" she asks.

"You are really, really 77-years-old," I confirm.

"That's not nice, D-D. You shouldn't tell me that."

"Alright, you're 37-years-old," I say.

"OK, now which is it? Am I 37-years-old or am I 77-years-old?" she presses on, missing my joke.

"Mom, you are 37 years old, but you look much younger." I shift gears.

"Good," she concludes. "Now D-D ... where's Fred?"

"He's at work," I fib. Kathy's had enough tears for today.

I find treating her disease with patience and humor helps her hold onto herself and not be ashamed of her confusion. If I can keep her rooted in her creative and hilarious potty mouth that still cracks everyone up ... I figure I can maximize our time as friends and as mother and daughter. While the disease progresses, I increasingly rely on lies to maintain balance amid her mental earthquake ("You have to shower because your sister's coming and you know how finicky she is"), but I know straight forward reasoning often makes the least sense to Kathy and causes her to be resistant.

You would think that the progression of Kathy's Alzheimer's would bring me down. And it does — I mean I'd much rather she not have Alzheimer's and we could spend time together shopping, enjoying ladies' luncheons, and yucking it up at the movies. But her story wasn't written that way. The fates gifted her with this progressive disease that only has one heart-wrenching ending. And yes, I'm often reduced to tears when nobody's looking, but I insist on keeping a stiff upper lip and fighting for her during this painful end. It's not easy, and even with all of the other family and caregivers, I often feel alone in the screeching pain of my mother's fears, ghosts and confusion. I have two brothers, but one of them lives in Albuquerque, and aside from the occasional stint up here to help, he's not here most of the time. And my second brother is her stepson and they've never had a great relationship, so he helps out in a pinch, but he doesn't have the inclination or ability to put his hands on this big rig. Since my father's death, I feel like Kathy and I are in a lonely bubble as she slides away and I struggle to hold on to her and give her the best life possible. I want this to be a time of fun, love, and even pride, but I would be lying if I told you it never brings me down.

And though I know I'm losing my mother one memory at a time, I stay right behind her and do everything in my power to help her enjoy what time she has left — and what time we have left together. And I know that she hasn't changed — it is her disease that's progressing. If I roll in sad and stressed, like a baby, my mom picks up on my vibe and she becomes sad and stressed. So I just don't do that. I bring her joy — and I get joy in return. It just makes everything so much better.

"Hey D-D," she continues.

"Yeah?"

"I'm dizzy," she tells me.

"I know Mom," I repeat. "Me too."

CHAPTER 2

Going home

"There's something I have to get off my chest," says a friend and burlesque performer, Waxie Moon, who's helping me with my next film. He appeared in my first documentary, and we've become close friends since then. On this new film about men who perform burlesque, Waxie's been my greatest cheerleader since I started working on the script. He and Jack and I are having breakfast at The Orleans casino during the yearly gala of burlesque, the Burlesque Hall of Fame, in Las Vegas. As Jack and I sit with Waxie over omelets and fruit plates to purr over the project, Waxie takes me in a completely different direction than I am expecting.

"I am so disappointed in your work on this project. You say you're going to call me back or email so-and-so and it just doesn't happen. If it does happen, it's so late that whatever task is at hand has lost its steam."

"Oh my God, honey, I'm so sorry," I scramble. It's true. While I've scaled the mountains of life with dogged enthusiasm, now I'm just tired. And forgetful. And confused. And increasingly dizzy. "I'm just kind of out of it lately. I'll get with the picture. I didn't think anybody noticed."

"Well, frankly, I noticed and I don't mean to be rude, but I've been shocked by your lack of progress."

I look at my tea. I don't know what to say. I have no explanation for how lame I've been over the past year. I look over at Jack, who's clearly having the same thoughts.

"I'm so sorry. There's something wrong. I just haven't been myself lately."

Waxie pays his tab and heads out after a humiliating meal.

"What is wrong with you?" Jack asks. "Sit up straight. You're all slumped over."

"I know," I say, squaring my shoulders and sitting up before slumping down seconds later.

On our flight home from Vegas, I feel hollow and embarrassed that yet another work trip has been a fruitless effort in getting this film off the ground.

"Honey, I think it's time we call Dr. F," I confess to Jack. I'm afraid Jack will think I'm committing the cardinal sin of being a lazy sack of shit. "Everything's just off. I'm not myself. The weight loss. The bruising. The dizziness. The confusion. The fatigue."

"I'm always tired too," Jack replies.

"That's just it!" I say. "I feel like a hypochondriac bugging the doctor about symptoms that everyone has. But I don't know, something feels epically wrong. I mean, I've been dizzy for more than a year now and it feels like it's getting worse by the day. I'm sorry. Am I being a hypochondriac? Shit. Maybe I am. Never mind."

"No, no, I'll email him tomorrow," he promises. "Want a martini?"

"No," I say. "I want two martinis."

"You look great," says my doctor. By now the bruises are gone and I'm feeling kind of silly sitting there in perfect health questioning my perfect health. "But just to be on the safe side, let's do an MRI."

"Well, since I have to pay for it, let me think about it," I answer. Because Jack works as a consultant, we decided years ago to opt for cheaper catastrophic insurance. We are, after all, a healthy family, and we reasoned why spend money on some schmancy insurance package that we wouldn't need? So I'm loath to spend money on any expensive tests because the first $10,000's on me.

I have a few friends who have also grappled with dizziness and they HIGHLY recommend a therapist at a Seattle clinic that specializes in balance disorders. I call the clinic on my way home from the doctor's office. They have an opening right now, so I turn the car around and head to the other side of town to meet with the exalted balance specialist.

After a series of coordination tests touching my pointer finger to my nose, walking while lifting my knees, taking a vision test, and completing a simple memory test, the dizziness specialist draws his conclusion.

"You have swelling on the right side of your brain, probably from PTSD," he assesses.

While it's true that life has had its challenges during the past four years — tending to my failing parents, seeing my father through his death, rearing Rose, all while trying to launch my next project and be a supportive spouse — a diagnosis of PTSD sounds squirrely. *I've just been living life*, I think. *It's not like I just finished a tour in Iraq or tried to smuggle my family into a safer country while dodging gunfire.* THOSE are *the people who get to claim PTSD. But just living life? Meh. I'm not convinced.*

"The good news is, it's not a brain tumor, and with dietary changes and physical therapy we can get rid of the dizziness," the balance specialists says.

"What about the fatigue and everything else?" I ask.

"As your dizziness eases, so should your other symptoms," he assures me.

His diagnosis doesn't sit right with me. PTSD? But he's so sure of himself that I feel, well, he must be right. Though he's not a doctor and he hasn't seen an MRI, he is so confident that I assume he must have seen this a million times and it's easy enough to accurately assess my condition with a handful of coordination tests. I mean, who am I to judge? He's no Joe Schmo, he's a bonafide balance pro.

He prescribes a diet high in dark leafy greens and low in processed carbohydrates and sugar. "Come back in a week and I think you'll notice a sizable change with these dietary changes."

On my way home, I look at the Reese's Peanut Butter Cup next to the driver's seat. It was going to be my afternoon treat.

I rip it open and eat it.

"I don't have brain cancer!" I tell Jack when I get home. I'm thinking, *Ha! Brain cancer? As if!* "I have PTSD from taking care of my parents and the inflammation it's causing in the right side of my brain dictates a low-sugar low-carb diet to get better. So *no mas vino y no mas tortillas.* Wah Wah Wah Waaaahhhh."

"That's probably good, I need to cut down on that stuff too. I'm craving vegetables anyway. This'll be good," he figures. "But PTSD, that's strange."

"I know, right?" I say. "Hey, do martinis have sugar?"

"I don't think so," he says.

"Then yes, please."

⊚ ⊚ ⊚

My daily routine is pretty set: take Rose — who's just finishing her junior year in high school — to school; walk the dogs; visit Kathy; pick Rose up from school; make dinner; eat dinner; clean up; tuck Rose in (who's usually doing homework in bed by now); drink martinis with Jack; and sack out in front of the TV. But as my dizziness grows, the routine falters. I ask Jack to drive Rose to school and pick her up. I opt for takeout and pizza more and more. I reduce doing the laundry and cleaning the house. Hell, I have maids come twice a month — I figure they can do all that. I start drinking less and sleeping more, sneaking naps when Kathy is snoozing and tucking in after bidding Rose good night. Where I used to work on scripts when I wasn't at my mom's, now I'm lucky if I squeeze out a few paltry emails about my movie every now and again.

Pinning my hopes on this new low-carb diet that will snap me out of my general funk, I'm disappointed as my constant sense of being drunk on a boat intensifies.

Like me, Kathy has lost a precipitous amount of weight over the past couple of months as *her* dizziness deepens. At night, she falls in her bedroom, fumbling around to execute her escape to 'go home.' Her latest fall has rendered her face into a bruised mass of purples, greens and yellows. Today, her gut is causing her so much pain that she cries in anguish.

"That's it," I tell one of her caregivers. "I'm taking her to the hospital."

Once we arrive at the hospital, it's determined that her potassium levels have bottomed out, probably from dehydration, even though we push water and electrolyte drinks on her constantly. The ER doctor determines that she should stay a couple of nights in the hospital so she can rehydrate and receive sorely lacking minerals in an IV drip. But see, Kathy can't really stay in the hospital restricted to a bed because she is now ALWAYS trying to 'go home.' I will have to stay with her or she will just tear out her IV and wander through the hospital, resisting help from the uniformed hospital staff while looking for an exit to home.

Exhausted, I lean over her ER bed railing to try to catch a nap as we wait for a doctor.

"Do you think if you fall asleep on the bed like that your noddle oddle diddle doodles will fall off and you'll fall over?" she asks me. Her speech has become very creative lately so we often play a little game of Guess What I Just Meant.

"You mean my arms?" I ask.

"Yeah, those," she says.

"I hope not," I say, eyes at halfmast.

Eventually, the ER nurse wheels her up to her room as I walk alongside her, holding her hand.

"Can you bring in a recliner chair so I can stay with her?" I ask.

"Sure thing," he says.

It's really not all that easy to keep an anxious Alzheimer's patient in a bed for a couple of days. Nope. Not easy at all. I draw on every distraction I can think of to keep her mind off her incarceration. We sing songs that I record on my iPhone. We take silly pictures on my iPhone and I filter them through funny apps. I try to get her to eat her cheese sandwiches and soup from the hospital's menu. I call people, begging them to visit us as a distraction. And at night, I jump up when she starts to stand and guide her into the bathroom.

The second night, I am so tired when she climbs out of the bed, I don't wake up. That is, until I hear liquid hitting the floor. I jump up.

"Mom, no no no no. You have to tinkle in the bathroom!"

Too late. She has left a sizable puddle at my now-wet feet and then crawls back into bed. I go into the hall and ask one of the night shift nurses if she can help me clean up the accident. She follows me with a bucket and a mop, curtly turning to my mom as she swabs the linoleum floor.

"You're supposed to pee in the toilet," she admonishes my mother before finishing and walking out the door.

Then, Kathy decides it's time to talk. And talk. And talk. I respond with grunts and mm-hmms.

"What time is it?" Kathy asks.

"One-thirty a.m.," I tell her.

"Why are we up so late?" she continues.

"Because you won't stop talking," I tell her.

Kathy laughs at that response. And so do I.

After a scant two hours sleep, the next morning Kathy's doctor visits.

"Kathy, you're looking good. Are you ready to go home?" he asks.

"Hell yes, I'm ready to go home," she tells him. "This place is a shithole."

"Deirdre, can you come with me to fill out her release forms?" he asks.

"Sure," I say, turning to my mom. "Stay here. OK? I'll be right back. Don't go anywhere, Mom."

"I won't," she promises.

"OK. Stay right there. I'll be right back," I reiterate.

When we get to the nurse's station, her doctor turns to me.

"I want Kathy released to a care center," he says. "We're getting too many ER visits with her, and the fact is, she needs 24-hour medical supervision now."

It's with sadness and relief that I hear his words. I'm finding it increasingly difficult to keep my mother contained in the house as her grip tightens on her fixation to "go home." Although the thought of an old-folks' home depresses me, I'm ready to release the task of guarding against falls, cleaning up incontinence-related accidents, feeding someone who doesn't want to eat, and trying to avert Kathy's overwhelming depression and boredom. Like a child, Kathy used to be happy — or at least distracted — if we turned on the TV (Fox News, hello!) and she ingested the video valium. Or I would give her a basket of rags and ask her to help me fold them. Or I would take her on a short walk. But none of that works anymore. She just sits in her chair by the window, refusing to eat and crying to go home. And though I always thought that the ultimate love I could provide her would be to keep her in her home forever, now I see that my mom needs to live in a community with a social life, 24-hour medical care, and alarms on the doors. While the not-so-little part of me is devastated because I know it's time to "put Mom in a home," it is so clearly the right thing to do.

Preparing for the inevitable, I've already been researching nursing homes for Alzheimer's patients. It's a painful process. Most places are secured with alarmed wings where patients graduate from retirement home, to assisted living, to lockup. There's often a chilling lack of windows or music in these wards, and cries and moaning punctuate the silence. Some places can't keep up with the patient load of incontinence and the acrid stench of soiled diapers stings the air. Other places boast about their food, where meatloaf looks like canned dog meat and vegetables are only recognizable because they're green or orange. No. It's not fun trying to find Mom's final home.

But the universe listens and I find a residence for dementia called Sunrise that is built like a five-star hotel. Overlooking downtown Mercer Island and Lake Washington, the vibe is homey. There are no white hallways with a single chair by a window that is bookended by locked doors. The rooms are like apartments. There are cushy seating areas and outdoor decks and constant sing-alongs and the air smells pleasant and the food actually looks and tastes like … food. When the residents cry to go home, the sweet staff comfort them with soft lies, like they're on a cruise that's pulling into harbor tonight and they'll be home soon.

It's where I'd want to go if I were in my mom's situation.

"Do you know where you'd like me to release her, or do you want to speak to a social worker?" her doctor asks.

"Let's get her into Sunrise. It's beautiful and it's like a home — not an asylum. She'll love it there. Or at least she won't hate it."

"Done," he says. "Let's get your mom home."

CHAPTER 3

From dingy to dreamy

I want to make Kathy's move into a nursing home as easy as possible. This isn't going to be easy, physically or mentally, for either of us.

I have so little strength; I have to outsource the operation. I hire movers to handle her furnishings. I look to my niece and nephew — who have been living in Seattle for the past year to help with my mother — to pack and schlep smaller items such as clothing, toiletries and lamps to her new home. I want to ask Jack or Rose to help, but Jack is completely sideswiped by work and compromised by a bad back, and Rose is fully swept up in finishing her junior year of high school and preparing for a summer trip to England. My brother Don, who lives in South Seattle and co-owns my father's company, is also too busy to help.

I bring my mom's finest furnishings from home and her favorite art and create a space that I hope will feel familiar to her. I only place a few family photos throughout her room because, frankly, she doesn't know who any of us are now. Perhaps to the irritation of the staff at her new home, I stay with Kathy every minute, sleeping on her sofa at night, for the first four nights. I just can't imagine leaving her, confused and upset that nothing is familiar to her in this new life.

"I wanna go home," Kathy repeats her endless loop.

"OK, I tell her," finessing my lies. "You just got out of the hospital and your doctor wants you to stay in this hotel until your meds are stable. But the good news is we're going home tomorrow."

"I was in the hospital?" she asks.

"Yes, but you're healthy now," I embellish and then redirect her. "Ready for dinner? There's a great restaurant down the street (downstairs)."

"Oh hell, I guess so," Kathy gives in.

Raised Mormon in Heber City Utah, Kathy grew up on snake, pheasant, deer and elk that her father hunted. Born in 1936 as the youngest of five children, she had a free spirit combined with the kind of charm that youngest children often have. As a child during WWII, she was scared shitless of a Nazi invasion and often recounted how frightening blackouts were and how impressive soldiers visiting home were. The war imbued her with a deep sense of national pride, and she was passionate about current world affairs. She also maintained a pioneer woman's attitude — strong as an ox and loaded with compassion. When she was a nurse and violent patients checked into her hospital, the staff would page the police ... and my mom. She could calm hysterical patients off any ledge, and when her negotiating skills failed, she could manhandle a 200-pound fighter back to bed with her signature brute strength and sympathetic grace. But her greatest gift, one which she still embraces in the thick of her disease, is her humor. She is part Lucille Ball, part Lily Tomlin, part Carol Burnett and always, ALWAYS (even now) wholly hilarious. My brother and I benefited from her intense drive and energy that drove her to work 70 hours a week so she could put us through private schools while my dad supported the house and paid for the groceries as an engineer.

But in 2005, she receded into herself, spending her days and nights in bed, occasionally wandering downstairs for a frozen dinner. She couldn't remember how to fry an egg. She couldn't remember how to get to her doctor's. More than once, she couldn't remember to open her garage door before backing her car out of the garage. She shut the world out, sequestering herself away to a corner bedroom at the end of a cul-de-sac on Mercer Island, hiding the embarrassment of her fading mind. The disease was sucking up her pioneer spirit, her tenacity as a world citizen, her convivial attitude, and her will to live.

"Mom, come on, let's go to lunch," I would implore.

"I can't," she would tell me, "I don't feel well."

"Why not? You never feel well," I'd beg. "Come on. What's the matter?"

"D-D, I just don't feel well," she'd tear up.

This went on for about a year. We tried Prozac. She wouldn't go to a counselor. I'd get her to my house for dinner on Sundays, but even seeing family didn't pull her out of her funk. It seemed hopeless. Finally (duh!), I thought to ask her what would help her get out of bed.

"A puppy," she said.

"Absolutely not," my dad emphatically responded. "I will not have a filthy beast in this house."

Fred wholeheartedly hated animals. While we had been allowed the occasional small dog or cat growing up, he was always resentful that somehow the 'beasts' had wormed their ways into our hearts and sullied our lives. In his childhood, there was no room for animals in a civilized home. His father, a Kansas state senator who died at 45 from a blood clot that traveled to his heart — had raised him formally, with proper grammar, elegant homes, a constant parade of the state's intelligentsia, and NO pets.

"Dad," I told him, "Mom's dying of depression. All she wants is a puppy. Getting one for her might get her out of bed. Period. End of discussion."

After that conversation, Fred finally acquiesced, approving the adoption of a puppy.

Kathy wanted a standard poodle. She had a black standard poodle in her 20s, and it was Kathy's favorite dog ever. Knowing I would probably inherit this dog some day, I felt poodles were too high-strung for me. But poodle mixes — Labradoodles, Goldendoodles, Schnoodles, German Shephoodles, Weimarnoodles, Whippletoodles, Pugoodles, Xoloitzcootles — a decent doodle mutt? I could live with that. Since doodles were so popular at the time, however, breeders had long waiting lists of eager adoptees willing to pay absurdly high prices for the little furry bundles of bouncing love. For months I fruit-lessly scoured the papers and searched online for a doodle for Kathy to no affordable avail.

One chilly day in 2006, a woman who ran a doodle puppy mill in Athol, Idaho, (that's right, "Asshole" with a lisp) chased her final ball to the sky, dumping more than 150 curly-headed bounders onto the rescue market. And so, Arthur, the seven-pound, eight-week-old, ginger-afroed, giardia-infected, mild-mannered, ball-obsessed, labra-doodlie-oodlie-oodlio came to be my mother's youngest child.

When I passed the puppy from my arms to hers, she cried tears of joy, pinching her own arm over and over, asking, "Is this a joke? If this is a joke, it's really mean, D-D, and I'll never forgive you. You have to tell me the truth. Is this a joke? Is he really mine?"

"It's no joke Mom, he's yours."

"But … your father!" she frowned, fearing that my dad would banish the small blur of energy.

"Dad said it's OK. The puppy is really, really yours," I promised. "So, what are you going to name him?"

"Arthur," she replied, without a moment's hesitation. "He looks just like my Uncle Arthur — frizzy red hair, beady eyes, and a big nose."

From that day on, Kathy rose early every morning from her well-worn king-sized cocoon as soon as her new bestie Arthur (whom she nicknamed "Curly") cried. She cleaned his accidents as if they were streams of silver and loaves of gold. She tromped around Mercer Island, bragging to her neighbors, her dental hygienists, her Albertson's cashiers, her longtime hair stylist, her Sav-On pharmacists, her Starbucks baristas — really to anybody who would follow her out to the parking lot to meet her pride and joy.

No longer a shut-in, Kathy spent the next six years smothering Mr. Arthur Doodle with her bounteous love. But as time worked its evil magic on Kathy, eventually she could no longer walk Arthur because of a bad hip (and if she did, she couldn't find her way home).

In her nursing home, my mother trips on a new pressing need beyond that of going home or finding my deceased father Fred. She has a new worry — the whereabouts of her labradoodle, Arthur.

"Where's Arthur?" she asks, over and over and over again.

"Laura's taking him for a walk," I lie. Clearly relieved for 15 seconds or so, Kathy looks at me and says, "Oh, good … Say, can you tell me where my dog is?"

With this latest shift in all of our lives, Kathy is not the only one who will have to settle into a new home. As Arthur cocks his head in confusion, I move his belongings (two dog beds, three leashes, and about 3,000 tennis balls) into my car and drive him to our home. Excited to be on a road trip, Arthur wags his tail and runs into our house, unknowingly losing one mom — but gaining another.

☉ ☉ ☉

"I want to show you this place I've found," Jack says, logging out of his computer where he's been working on an Excel spreadsheet for a client.

"A place for what?" I ask.

"For a barbecue joint," he says.

"Wow, OK," I say, somewhat surprised that he has been seriously considering opening a restaurant even though we have only mused on the topic to date. "Is it open? We could go now?"

"Yeah," he says, grabbing his car keys.

We drive to a dingy sports bar that is long past its expiration date in Seattle's industrial Sodo district. The bar's pungent aroma approximates a heady combo of urine, vomit, excrement, smoke and booze. Pull tabs anchor the bar and large screen TVs adorn every wall and hide the windows. Random chain-link fences define the large space's interior for a stage, a pool table, a bar and a dining area. Black composite board covers the windows in an upstairs bar that was allegedly used for nefarious activities.

It is, in a word, odious. But as repugnant as I find it, the place is packed with workers from the area having a beer, watching a football game, and having a hell of a good time.

"And you like this place because?" I ask Jack.

"Because it's big, it has a parking lot, it's not in a family neighborhood so I can smoke here, and did I mention it has a big parking lot?"

"Yeah, you said that," I answer, incredulous at how grim the place is. "Look, there's nothing around here but warehouses — and your parking lot."

"Which is perfect!" he carries on. "There are no local residents, so the smoke won't bother them. There is nowhere for all the workers around here to eat. And there's parking! We could kill it at lunchtime."

"And dinner?" I ask. "You think people are actually going to get in their cars, drive to an industrial zone where the only foot traffic is homeless people? Not to mention there's no established dining scene in this ... neighborhood." The people sitting around us collectively scream when someone scores a touchdown on one of the many TVs.

"Yes?" he hesitates.

"Another round?" the bartender yells above the crowd.

"I think I better," I yell back.

"Sure," Jack says, turning to me.

"Whaddya think?" he asks. "It has an offer pending, but if that falls through maybe I could get funding to buy it."

"Where would you get that money?" I ask. I'm all for Jack chasing a dream and I don't want to cock-block his artistic journey, but I'm just not seeing it here.

"I don't know," he admits. "I'll just start calling my friends in high-tech."

"OK, well," I say, not wanting to sound like a party pooper. "I say, go for it."

"I will," he says, looking around the dank hellhole with stars in his eyes.

CHAPTER 4

The bliss of ignorance

I'm back for my second session at the dizziness clinic.

"How are you feeling?" asks my therapist.

"I don't know … the same … worse?" I answer.

"And you followed the no-sugar diet? You know, sugar causes inflammation and is doubtless contributing to the swelling in the right side of your brain," he surmises.

"Yes. I followed the diet," I tell him. And outside of the Reese's Peanut Butter Cup a week ago, I did follow the diet. I hate chard, but I ate it dammit.

"Good," he responds. "We're gonna add physical therapy now."

After more laborious tests of walking in a straight line and touching my elbow to my knee or looking left as I walk straight or doing deep knee bends as if I work in the Bureau of Funny Walks, he prescribes a series of daily exercises. I take that list with me and drive to the store to do my grocery shopping. In the Safeway parking lot, I run into a pylon while parking. It seems like I hit it in slow-motion.

"What happened to the fender?" Jack asks, noticing the damage when I get home.

"Sorry sweetie," I answer, too exhausted to feel truly apologetic for the dent. "I hit a pylon at Safeway. Just ran right into it while parking."

God dammit, I can see him thinking.

"I thorry," I say, assuming my kicked-puppy look widening my eyes and lowering my head.

"Oh well, I guess this isn't the end of life as we know it," he forgivingly says.

When I return to the balance therapist a week later (having consumed not a whiff of sugar), I am, if anything, dizzier.

"OK, let's see what we're working with this week," says the therapist. "I want you to walk on this line, heel to toe and heel to toe."

"Like in a sobriety test?" I ask. I wish I hadn't said that. Like, that's my first association.

"Yes. Like in a sobriety test."

And … I can't do it. It's 9 in the morning, and I can't pass a basic sobriety test. I look at the therapist and think, *Shit, I have 59 more minutes with this yahoo and I just want to go home, lie down, and go to sleep.*

"Now, follow my finger with your eyes … Now with just your right eye … Now with just your left eye …,"

As I'm driving home with my latest assignment of home exercises, I call Jack on my cell.

"Yeah, no. I don't think this therapy is working. I'm just not buying it," I say. "Can you email our doctor? I think it's time for that MRI.

I'm sorry. I hate to spend the money, honey, but I can barely drive, let alone walk now."

"Done," says Jack.

Later that week I greet the receptionist at Seattle Radiology. "I believe you are going to take pictures of my brain today," I say light-heartedly.

"Here you are," she says, looking at her computer. "If you could fill out this form, we'll call you shortly."

"Fab," I say, taking the clipboard holding a small novel of forms.

Pregnant? No.

Trying to get pregnant? God no.

Major surgeries? Yes! C-section when Rose was born.

Diabetes? No.

Heart disease? No.

Cancer? Certainly not.

I check off the list of noes. My dad used to love introducing me to people in a heavy Eastern Bloc accent, declaring, "This is my daughter, Dee-drah. She's strong like bull, make good baby."

And here I sit, looking out over Seattle's skyline from the clinic's 11th floor office proudly checking off all the noes in the form. *Strong like bull, make good baby.*

"Deirdre Timmons?" calls a tech in blue scrubs.

"Bingo!" I stand.

As the technician walks me back he asks me how I am.

"If I were any better it would be a crime," I joke.

"Great! I love that," he says. "Ever had a brain MRI?"

"I had a couple for my neck for a herniated disc years ago. Lovely experience," I joke again.

"So you know. It's loud and you have to hold still and all that?"

"Oh, I know," I say.

"Here's your robe. Take off all your jewelry. You don't have any metal such as a pacemaker or shrapnel do you?"

"Oh no, they got all the shrapnel out after my tour in 'Nam."

"Funny! OK, come on out when you're dressed. We're ready for you," he says.

I step out onto the cold floor in my fashionable hospital attire. Brrrr.

"Let's have you jump on that bed and scooch all the way up till your head is here," he says, pointing at a plastic headrest. "Here's the panic button, press it three times if you need us to take you out."

Ew. I look at the tube. I hate the tube. I feel like I become human sausage in a metal casing in the tube. "You know what?" I ask, "I'm freezing. Can I have a blanket and can you cover my eyes so I don't have to see all this?"

"Sure thing," replies the tech, draping me in a thin warmed blanket and placing a dry washcloth over my eyes. "OK, I'm heading out now. This should take about 40 minutes. Enjoy."

"Oh, you can rest assured I will enjoy this."

For the next 40 minutes, it sounds like I'm in the center of a construction zone at a hospital. The sirens and clanks and banging and ringing are deafening. It is, in a word, unpleasant.

"Good job, Deirdre," the tech says on the loudspeaker. "We're gonna pull you out now."

As I slide out of the suffocating metal tube, the tech has shed his lighthearted demeanor.

"So, what'd ya see?" I goad.

"Are you seeing your doctor today?" he asks.

"I wasn't planning on it," I say. "Why? Should I? Wait! Did you see something?"

"I don't read them," he hesitates. "You'll have to talk to your doctor."

That's an odd reaction, I think. *Where's my happy tech from 40 minutes ago?*

"Okaaay. See ya later, NOT!" I tease.

As I drive home, my cell rings. I scan the road for cops, then pick up.

"Herro."

"Deirdre, it's Seth," says my doctor.

"Hey Seth, whazzzuuuup?" I ask.

"Where are you now?" he asks.

"Driving home. I just left the MRI place."

"Is there any chance you can turn around and come back for a second MRI now?" he asks.

"No, sorry. I have to pick up Rose at school."

"How about tomorrow morning? Can you come in then for a second MRI?" he asks.

"No, I'm busy all day. But I can come in day after tomorrow," I tell him. "Why? Is something wrong?"

"I wanna do a second MRI with contrast," he says. "The first one is too fuzzy."

"Oh, then yeah, I'll come back day-after-tomorrow," I agree.

"Great. My nurse will call you with your appointment," he says. "Have a good evening and say hi to Jack and Rose for me."

"Oba-kayba. *Ciao*."

"Bye Deirdre."

The second MRI is much like the first, only this time I get an IV that pumps contrast dye into my veins so they can see different parts of my brain more clearly.

"Deirdre," says the MRI tech into my headphones, "I need you not to swallow for the next five minutes while we look at your neck."

"Gotcha!" I yell back. I don't know if I have to yell or if there's a mic on me or what, but I figure they're in a whole different room so it can't hurt if I raise my voice a little.

Now listen, lying on your back and not swallowing for five minutes is akin to some wartime torture. The first 30 seconds are no big deal, but then the spit starts collecting at the back of your throat, and the more it collects, the more spittle your mouth makes until your mouth is half-full of saliva and you HAVE to swallow or you'll drown. And then JUST when you think you're drowning, the tech says, "Good job. You can swallow now. We're just gonna do that a few more times."

"How was it?" he asks, sliding me out of the tube.

"It sucked!" I say quite honestly. "That no-spitting business is for the birds! No joke, I thought I was going to drown."

"I know," he sympathizes. "Sorry about that. But your pictures are great, crystal clear. So … good job even if it was terrible. Are you seeing your doctor after this?"

"Oh, yeah, I have an appointment with him now," I remember. Thank God the tech reminded me or I would have totally forgotten and driven straight home.

I go down the elevator, across the entry, into the adjacent high-rise, and up another elevator. Having been built and rebuilt over a span of 100 years on Seattle's First Hill, Swedish Medical Center is a complicated skein of buildings and tunnels and breezeways and elevators and lobbies. I'm pretty much always lost here.

As I enter my doctor's office, I immediately relax. Dr. F has been our family doctor since forever. Before he treated our family, he completed part of his residency with my mother while she was the night charge nurse at the Boeing Clinic. They became close friends during that time, and as he shifted from family friend to family doctor, we all still felt great familial affection for him.

After the nurse checks my vitals and asks how life is going, Dr. F comes barreling in full of good cheer.

"Hi, Deirdre," he says, giving me a big bear hug. "What's going on?"

"God, right?! This dizziness is out of control," I tell him. "Are you seeing anything on the MRIs?"

"Well, we don't know," he answers tentatively. "Something is definitely there, we just don't know what it is. All we know is it's a dense mass in your brain. At first I thought you might have sarcoidosis, which is an inflammatory disease that can affect the heart and major organs. But seeing this mass, we're looking at the possibility of MS, but it's not consistent with typical MS scans. It could be a tumor. It could be from a stroke."

"What does the radiologist think?" I ask, feeling strangely removed from his words, like we're talking about someone else.

"He's not sure. He's sending your scans to a radiology conference tomorrow to see if a more extended network of radiologists can identify it," he says.

"Oh," I say. I'm sort of proud of my dense brain mass — it's going to a conference and it's only a couple of days old. "So what's next?"

"I'd like to do a heart X-ray and some blood tests next, just so we can start ruling out possibilities," says Dr. F.

"OK." I feel like I'm watching a TV show and the good-looking doctor is trying to unravel a complicated medical challenge.

He doesn't waste any time. Before I leave, the nurse takes chest X-rays, the phlebotomist draws vials of my blood, and the front desk makes an appointment for a CAT scan of my major organs. The next 24 hours are spent working through the hospital maze, putting gowns on, taking gowns off, stopping at Starbucks in the hallways for a chai latte or a breakfast sandwich, checking in, checking out, getting poked with needles and dressed in lead aprons for the various scans. I feel like this is a whole lot of fuss over some insipid little problem that the doctors will ultimately declare is dehydration, maybe, or a dearth of some important vitamin. Never having grappled with any serious health concerns, I flitter hither and thither mindlessly, allowing the medical professionals to poke and prod at me in their little game of Operation.

Dr. F's office calls me sometime during all the testing.

"Hi, Deirdre, this is Cindy at Dr. F's office," the sweet voice coos.

"Hi, Cindy."

"Do you have time for a quick MRI of your liver tomorrow morning?" she asks. "We found something irregular in your CAT scan and we just want to double check it."

"OK," I say, actually nervous for the first time since this whole thing started. If I have cirrhosis of the liver from years of — shall we say — slightly excessive celebration, I'm going to be so embarrassed. I will not be able to call everyone and say, "Yeah, because I'm such a big ol' lush, I now have liver cancer. Nice, huh?"

The next morning, I go in for my liver MRI. By now, I know half the staff at Seattle Radiology.

"Hey," I greet today's tech.

"I see we're doing your liver today," he says.

"Yeah, apparently there was something dodgy about that area in one of the tests," I admit. "Can I ask you something?"

"Sure," he says.

He was the very first technician I saw who had been so cheerful before my MRI, and then so sober after my MRI.

"Did you see the mass in my brain that first day?" I ask. "You can be honest because I know about it now."

"Yeah," he admits. "We saw it."

"Why didn't you tell me?" I ask.

"That's not my job," he answers.

"Do you think you know what this is?" I ask.

"No."

"Well, if you see anything in this MRI on my liver, will you tell me?" I ask. "As a favor?"

"No," he says. "Again, not my job."

Damn, I think. People and their professional professionalism!

CHAPTER 5

The end of the world as we know it

"Hi, Mom. It's your daughter Deirdre," I say bending down, kissing my mother on the cheek while pulling two Snickers out of my pocket. "Look what I brought you."

"What is it?" she asks.

"Reese's," I tell her, grinning.

"What's that?" she asks.

"Only one your favorite candies," I sing, ripping it open. "Here you go. Good, but not good for you."

"Oh, thank you honey," she says taking the candy bar. "Where's Arthur?"

"Laura's taking him for a walk," I lie. I usually try to bring Arthur when I visit Mom in her new digs, but today I didn't have time what with my latest adventures in sterile hallways and rooms. "She's taking him to poop, then they'll be back."

"Oh good," she replies.

"Hey," Joan, one of the dementia residents says. She is sitting next to Kathy in the living room. An old movie is playing on the very-big-screen TV. The room is about half full with residents — some in wheelchairs, some in chairs or on sofas. About half the people are asleep. The other half sit quietly, looking neither here nor there. I don't think anyone's watching the movie.

"I want one of those," says Joan.

Dammit. I forgot to sneak my mom upstairs before giving her a treat. Three or four people are now looking at me, or, at the other Reese's in my hand.

"Give me one of those," Joan persists.

"OK," I say. "Let me go get you one. Mom, come on, let's go upstairs and get one for everyone."

"Get one what?" she asks.

"A cookie," I say, calling the candy bar a cookie because Kathy still seems to understand that cookies are sweet and she likes sweet. So anything called a 'cookie' she likes.

"I want a cookie," Joan almost yells.

"Me too," says my mom.

"You already have one," I tell my mom.

"Have one what?" she asks.

"A cookie!" I say, kind of curtly. I usually don't mind the repetition and redirection of being with my mom, but today I'm just not in the mood. Today I just want to tell her all I've been going through and hear her wise nurse's thoughts, even though that wisdom only lives in my memory now.

"I want one!" Joan reiterates.

"I know, Joan, we'll get you one," I promise, ushering my mom away while more eyeballs turn accusingly toward us. "We'll get one for everyone."

"Get what for everyone?" my mom asks.

"You'll see … just … come on." We amble to a seating enclave down the hall and out-of-view of the group family room as Joan yells toward us, "Bring me my cookie!"

"Now, about those candy bars," I remind Kathy.

"What candy bars?" she asks.

"The one in your hand," I say, holding up her hand with the candy bar in it.

"Oh, where'd I get that?" she asks.

"I brought it," I remind her. "D-D, your daughter."

"I know who you are," she says defensively (and unconvincingly). "My beautiful daughter. You look great. Have you lost weight?"

"Yes," I tell her. This is a conversation I don't mind repeating because even though I'm so thin now that it hurts to sit on any hard surface, I love, LOVE being model thin. And my mother — who had me on extreme diets my entire childhood — is the perfect audience to admire my newly lithe frame. "I've been losing weight and the doctors don't know why. So they're doing a bunch of tests to figure out why I'm losing weight."

"Well," she says, setting me up for a joke. "While you're seeing all these doctors, have them do something about that nose."

Kathy's always been a physically attractive woman. As grounded and tough as she was, her good looks were of tantamount impor-tance to her. And being a caring mother with hope for her daughter's success in her heart, she extended her dedication to beauty by trying to maximize what flawed looks I had. She started by spritzing lemon in my hair as a toddler to make sure I had sun-kissed blonde hair. As I aged, the hair treatments progressed from lemon, to Sun-In, to frosting my hair, and ultimately, to bleaching it. She saw to it that I was a true blonde and I'd have the historical photos to prove it. And more than once, she jokingly hinted that I might want to look into getting a nose job. It was one of those recurring jokes that increasingly caused me to wonder, "Should I get a nose job?"

She was so charismatic, funny, smart and convincing, that I grew up believing the Kathy Mantra: You can never be too rich or too thin. Even now, not a day goes by that I don't henpeck my physicality and fixate on some perceived imperfection. With the help of maturation (and many Oprah articles), I've made some peace with my bloops and sags and lines, but I have my moments … often.

When Kathy realized her observations about my physicality no longer bugged me, her advice and admonishments took on a humorous angle and her criticisms evolved into good-hearted banter, calling out her criticisms in the form as a joke. But don't hate. I love how she teases my looks now and I'm just happy that her biting humor has survived. Deep in the jokes of her comical criticism lies the woman who no longer recognizes me, but on some level, still sees me.

"How are your parents?" she asks.

"Well, you're my mother," I tell her.

"So, how are your parents?" she repeats.

"Well, you're my mother, so you're my parent," I explain. "How are you?"

"Wait, you're mine?" she points at me.

"I'm your daughter, Deirdre," I say.

"Oh, how embarrassing," she says, "I'm sorry, D-D."

"It's OK. If you're gonna make that mistake, you might as well make it with me."

"So, who's your father?" she continues working out the puzzle.

"Fred."

"He is?" she asks, cocking her head.

"Yup."

"I thought we just had those two awful boys," she says, with a deep look of consternation. "You don't look like my daughter."

"Well," I tell her, "I looked different when I was born."

"How can I be so stupid?" she asks.

"You're not stupid," I explain. "You have Alzheimer's."

"Did I call you D-D when you were little? I love that name. 'Hey, D-D. Hey little D-D,'" she acts out her revelation. "I just thought you were a nice kid who came here. I thought, Wow! She comes here and helps out. How nice. Boy, Arthur sure likes you. I sure like you too. Well, did I raise you?"

"Yup."

"What do you go by?" she asks.

"D-D."

"So, who was your mom?" she presses on.

"You," I tell her.

"Why?" she asks.

"Because you're my mom."

"I don't remember it," she confesses.

"Yup. I'm your daughter. You can't escape it."

"I wouldn't want to," she says. "Did you ever get married?"

"Yup," I say. "I married Jack."

"Oh, that's right. Jack is on the loose," she says, narrowing her eyes. "So, what's your first name?"

"Deirdre."

"Yeah, that's right," she says, grasping the story for a fleeting moment. "Don't tell Fred this."

"It would be hard to tell him," I say. "He died a couple of months ago."

"Oh then," she says, laughing. "Go ahead and tell him."

At home, nothing's different. I don't really clean up much or make dinner. I make anemic attempts to work on my film, but after I walk the dogs I'm tuckered out for the rest of the day. I can barely pull it together to drop Rose off at school every morning and pick her up from school every afternoon. I feel like I'm one of the laziest people I know and wonder when I started being so lazy. I didn't used to be lazy. Or, I don't think I was.

Oh well. Ellen's on in 20 minutes so I'll just relax until then. I've never been a TV watcher, except maybe when I was in elementary school and "Gilligan's Island" and "I Dream of Genie" and "The Six Million Dollar Man" pretty much dominated my world. But that was a long time ago. When did I start watching TV again? Hmmm.

My cell rings like a church bell.

"Herro!" I say, recognizing my doctor's number. "Oregon State Prison."

"I'm sorry?" says Dr. F.

"Just kidding. *C'est moi*, Deirdre," I tell him.

"Hello Deirdre! Can you talk now?"

"I don't know. Jack's not around. I think we're safe," I say in a ridiculously over-the-top sexy voice.

"Ha," he says. "So, we are looking at the data we've collected on you and we still don't know what that mass is in your right cerebellum."

"An alien?" I ask.

"I don't think so," he puts up with me. "I am talking to a group of radiologists and other people in the field and we're all a little stumped by your case."

"Maybe it's a whole pod of aliens?" I offer.

"And again, no," he says. "Normally we would proceed to a lumbar puncture to see if there's anything in your spinal cord that would help us solve the mystery. But what I want to do next is send you to a neurologist to have her look at your tests before we subject you to a spinal tap. Are you free tomorrow at 3?"

And so I book yet another appointment. And I wait yet another night, telling Jack that even five days into this laborious testing, we still have no answers, and blah blah blah.

"Do you want me to go with you to the neurologist?" he offers.

"God no," I tell him. "There's no use in both of us wasting time on this."

I have become a pro in the testing world. I stride up to the receptionist with driver's license, insurance card and parking ticket (for validation) in hand. I call out my name, time of appointment, and doctor I'm seeing or procedure I'm having. I fill out my forms, though slowly, since it's becoming increasingly difficult for me to write by hand. I turn everything in, grab a magazine, and settle in till I hear …

"Deirdre!?"

"That is I!" I declare, playing the familiar game.

"The doctor is ready to see you."

"And I am ready to see her," I proclaim to the good nurse.

We march back, away from the waiting room, through a mass of hallways. I'm invited into a little room. The nurse flies the plastic flag that indicates patient present. The nurse takes my vitals and then she bids me adieu. I look around the room. I pull out my phone. It gets no reception. I look back around the little room. I cross my legs. I uncross my legs. I shiver. It's cold in here even though it's late June. I recross my legs. I exhale loudly. This room has no magazines. Bummer. An efficient-looking, quite serious woman enters. I do not make any jokes. She has me touch my left finger to my nose and then she has me touch my right finger to my nose. The right side is oddly challenging. She has me run my left heel down my right shin and then she has me run my right heel down my left shin. This is new — I can't control my right heel. She has me follow her finger with my right eye, then she has me follow her finger with my left eye. My right eye moves in stop-motion, not fluidly. She gives me the sobriety test, heel-to-toe, heel-to-toe. I teeter and can't do it. She invites me to walk up and down the hall. I pass with flying colors. She kindly brings me back into the small room where I spell words backwards, most of them unsuccessfully. She pulls up my MRIs on her computer. She turns to me.

"It's time for a brain biopsy."

"Wow," I tell Jack when I get home. "This is beginning to feel for real."

He sits in his IKEA office chair where he works from home and listens to my update.

"A biopsy?" he asks, surprised. "What do they think it is?"

I shrug. "Nobody seems to know. They want to collect a brain sample. An actual honest-to-god chunk of my brain."

"I'm calling Dr. F," he says resolutely.

"No, don't bug him," I argue. "I have an appointment tomorrow morning. I'll ask him what he really thinks is going on.

"Can you write down what he says?" asks Jack, who can't go to the morning's appointment because he has a business meeting. "I don't want you to forget what he tells you."

"Oh God," I say, exasperated. Like I'm too dumb to go to my own appointments. "I won't forget. Sheesh. I'm not a child, you know."

"Yeah, well, you forget a lot of things lately," he hesitates.

"I'll take notes!" I say, rolling my eyes. "Promise. Cross my heart hope to die."

When I get to the doctor's office the next morning, a nurse enters and takes my vitals.

"I have a question for you, Deirdre," the nurse says.

"Shoot," I say.

"Do you have a good support network at home?" she asks.

"I guess so," I answer, wondering what that actually means.

"Good. Also," she continues, "do we have a living will on file for you?"

"I have one, but I don't think you guys have a copy of it," I tell her.

"If you could just have someone fax it to us, that would be great," she says.

"OK," I say, thinking our lawyer can do that. Then thinking, *That's odd. Why would they want my living will on file? Do-wha?*

The nurse sweeps out of the room shortly before Dr. F enters.

"Hello Deirdre," he warmly greets me. "So, we're still stumped by the mass in your brain. We have ruled out sarcoidosis, MS and a stroke, which leaves us thinking it may be some sort of tumor, but again, we're not sure. At this point, we believe it would be best to collect a sample of the mass to determine exactly what it is, which is why the neurologist suggested a brain biopsy."

In my heart of hearts, I know it's not a brain tumor, so I ignore the mention of it. After all, there is NO history of cancer in my family, so I don't even acknowledge that he's said that scary word. At this point, I'm pretty sure my diagnosis is going to be Alzheimer's. Not that that doesn't scare me … but I'm confident a cure for Alzheimer's is just around the corner and I'll be able to skirt the disease with medical innovations.

"Aye-aye Captain," I say, imagining they're going to sink a needle deep into my brain to extract some brain cells.

It's been more than a week since this hullabaloo began, and if a quick needle poke can solve the mystery, then we can all set our sights on stopping the dizziness and focus on addressing my probable Alzheimer's. After another MRI to map my brain, I visit the brain surgeon to prep for tomorrow's procedure. In fact, the very same brain surgeon who twice injected steroids into my neck for my herniated disc years ago is going to do my biopsy. Somehow, that fact strikes me as odd.

The surgeon pulls out a pen and starts drawing on my forehead.

"What's that for?" I ask.

"We have to map where we're putting the head brace for the surgery," she explains, putting down the pen and pulling out an electric razor.

"Whoa, what's that for?" I ask.

"I'm going to shave the hair where the incision will be made and where the screws will anchor."

"Whoa whoa whoa, wait a minute. What screws?" I hold up my hand.

"The screws that will anchor the skull brace so you can't move during the procedure," she says matter-of-factly.

Screws? Skull brace? These words don't sound good to me. Dr. F didn't warn me of this.

"You're shaving my head and drilling screws into my head?" I check.

"Yes," she says.

"Wait," I have to digest this. "Do you have to shave my hair?"

"Yup," she says lightheartedly.

Fuck. FUCK.

"OK," I say. "I guess it'll grow back."

"Yes," she says again. "Hair grows back."

"Wait," I

I hold my hand up again. "Can you just shave tiny spots?"

And then, she looks at me, as if to say, 'Girl, this is just the beginning. Get over it,' and she turns on the razor.

I look at the exam table as small strands of hair fall on the paper liner. She then attaches two stickies with snaps to my temples, before — brace yourself — before NAILING them into my head. OK, they're teeny tiny nails, but she NAILS the stickies with snaps, I repeat, she NAILS the stickies with snaps into my head! No warning. No, "Hey, I'm about to nail your head." She just nails me.

"Ow!" I quite appropriately exclaim.

"Just one more," she breezily says.

God, I wish Jack — or anybody — were here in this room with me to witness this medieval torture. "This is where we'll enter the skull to gain access to the right cerebellum where the swelling is."

"Don't you just draw a sample through a hypodermic needle?" I ask.

"No," she says matter-of-factly. "We take a plug of skull out and cut into the brain to acquire the sample."

I don't know what to say to that. In fact, I think it's safe to say that I go into a little state of shock with this explanation.

"Oh," is all I can muster.

The brain surgeon finishes drawing on me, shaving me, NAILING me, and chirps, "OK. I'll see you tomorrow morning."

The following morning I sit in the surgery staging area where patients rest in hospital-style (read: bodily-fluid resistant Naugahyde) reclining chairs.

"Would you like a heated blanket?" asks the prep nurse.

"Yes I would," I say, chilly in my gown and rubber-treaded hospital socks. Jack sits next to me sipping coffee. I would love a coffee right about now. It's 6 in the morning and I can barely keep my eyes open. But they don't want me throwing up and choking on my vomit and dying while under sedation — so I haven't been able to eat or drink anything since last night. The tech returns with two of those heavenly heated blankets. "The anesthesiologist is on his way."

"Hello, I'm Dr. Z, and I'll be your anesthesiologist today."

"Hello, I'm Deirdre," I respond. "I'll be your patient today."

After discussing drugs and the procedure that I don't really hear because it's 6 a.m. in the morning with no coffee, he asks, "Is there anything I can get you?"

"A martini?" I ask.

"Sorry, we don't have any of those," he laughs. "Are you anxious?"

"Should I be?" I ask. I mean, I didn't love the thought of this morning's activity, but I certainly wasn't anxious until he asked me that. Up until now, I was just thinking I was in the hands of pros and there was no reason to worry.

"Well, many people are anxious before brain surgery," he says.

"This is just a brain biopsy," I explain to him. And then I think, *Shit, this is brain surgery. I'm about to have brain surgery. It's not just going to be a needle sunk deep in my brain to take out a few cells. They're taking out a plug of my skull and going to the center of my brain and removing a chunk of it. This isn't a quick teriyaki lunch. This. Is. Brain. Surgery.*

"Sometimes people like anti-anxiety medication before procedures," the anesthesiologist continues.

"But, my 'procedure' is in, like, 10 minutes," I point out. "Would an anti-anxiety pill even have time to take effect before I go in?"

"Probably not," he agrees.

"Thanks, but I think I can handle it," I tell him. "I'm actually not nervous."

"OK," he says. "I'll see you soon then."

I'm eventually wheeled into pre-surgery, where the anesthesiologist swings by carrying a hypodermic needle. *Shit*, I think, *another poke*. But I'm spared the prick and he pumps a liquid straight into my IV tube.

And my world goes black.

I don't know how long I've been asleep, but I wake myself up bellowing some sort of primal wail. My head feels like a large wooden ball. I have no thoughts — at least that I'm aware off. But the sound coming out of my mouth is like something I've never heard from me or anyone else. I feel like I'm floating in a place I've never been before. I can sense Jack near me. I can sense his worry. But I can't open my eyes, nor can I stop the sound I'm making.

Someone enters our curtained-off alcove.

"What's going on?" Jack asks urgently. He sounds so far away.

"It's probably the drugs she's coming off and the trauma she's been through," says someone. My right arm tightens as they take my blood pressure. I feel a swipe of the thermometer across my forehead. A clamp is attached to my left pointing finger to read my oxygen levels. I know this intuitively because I've had it done so many times recently. "We'll take her up to a private room where she can recuperate."

In a blur of doors and hallways and ramps and elevators, I keep my eyes mostly closed as I continue to wail in … what … realization that something has shifted? That my brain has been violated and the information that that procedure contains is going to change my life? That I am now in very real danger?

In the distance, I feel my bed moved through a doorway to what I know is my hospital room. Again with the vitals.

"We'll give her something to relax," another voice says.

"Is she … OK?" asks Jack, speaking through a long tunnel.

"She'll be fine," says the voice. "She'll go to sleep now."

And then, all voices recede back into a pipe and everything goes quiet.

When I open my eyes, Jack is sitting next to me. He leans in, looking pretty freaked out.

"Hi," he gravely says. He stands up and kisses my cheek. "How do you feel?"

"Oh," I say. I don't know how to describe how I feel because I've never felt this way before. "I don't know."

"You were really messed up when you came out of it," he says.

"I know. I was wailing or something, wasn't I?"

"Yeah you were. You had me worried."

"I'm OK," I say. "Just dizzy. And my skull feels weird. Where's Rose?"

"She went home with Hadley," he explains. Hadley is one of Rosemary's oldest friends.

"Is she coming here?" I ask him.

"Do you want her to?"

"I don't know," I say. "I'm pretty messed up. Maybe she shouldn't see me like this."

"She's staying the night at Hadley's house," he says.

I'm staying the night at the hospital and this makes no sense.

"No no no no no. I want you to go home to her tonight," I say.

"OK, whatever you want," he says.

"After we talk to the doctor, go home and be with her. I'm just going to sleep tonight," I reason.

"Can I get you anything?" he asks.

"No, thank you." And I go back to sleep.

When I wake up it's late afternoon. My brother- and sister-in-law, Jim and Libby, are in the room.

"Hi," says Libby, reaching down to hug me.

"Hi," I answer.

"Hi D-D," Jim steps in, hugging me. "We heard it was quite an ordeal."

"Yeah," I say.

"What a beautiful view," Libby comments, looking out of the large window that overlooks Seattle's Capitol Hill and a beautiful old church on the hill. I'm facing away from the window so I can't see the view.

"How do you feel?" asks Libby, genuinely concerned.

"I don't know," I answer honestly. "I just had my head cracked open."

We all kind of laugh. Kind of.

A delivery of gourmet sandwiches from my friend Monica shows up.

"Party at the Timmons'!" I joke.

Nobody's really hungry, but I implore them to eat.

The nurse enters and takes my vitals. Jack introduces her to Jim and Libby and they ask her a number of questions that she can't answer.

"The doctor will be in tonight to tell you how the operation went," she tells them. "She'll probably be here in a couple of hours."

After the nurse leaves, there's a lull in this party.

"Why don't you guys go to Jimmy's and get a martini?" I suggest, referring to the martini bar a block away.

"We don't want to leave you," they all say. But I can tell that that notion is a welcome idea. Shoot, I'd go with them if I could.

"I want to sleep," I assure them. "Go for me. The doctor won't be here for a while anyway."

They leave, and I recede into the comfort of slumber.

My posse returns just as I'm waking up. The nurse returns and asks if we need anything. We don't, but Jack asks her if the results of my biopsy are in. It's early evening now.

"Your doctor will be here soon to discuss them, but I'd be happy to pull up Deirdre's chart to see if the results are in," she says, typing into the room's computer. "Oh, yeah, they're here!"

Jack steps over to the computer and has a look. He returns to my side and sits silently. I assume no news is good news. But, he's uncharacteristically quiet. After 20 minutes or so, I turn to him.

"Did the report say something?" I ask. "You're so quiet."

"Yes," he says, beginning to tear up. "It says you have a malignant brain tumor." He takes my right hand and sobs into it.

For the first time in my life, I can't think of anything funny to say.

It seems like an eternity before the doctor arrives. I'm not crying. I'm not talking. None of us are. We are completely muted by the information. In fact, I feel like this all has nothing to do with me and I am just a witness in a corner of the room watching this woman surrounded by loved ones who are in a silent panic. The woman in the bed is not me. She is a character with a malignant brain tumor who's in a lot of trouble.

"Hi," the surgeon says upon entering the room.

"Hi," I say back. I don't want to hear what she has to say.

"Well, the good news is, your biopsy was a success," she says smiling. "The bad news is you have a fast-growing inoperable brain tumor called a medulloblastoma in your right cerebellum. There is no cure, but we will try to turn a month into a year or two. But again, there is no cure." We are all silent. "I'm sorry. You just drew the short straw."

Jack holds my hand and stares blankly at her. Libby's hand is at her mouth. Jim can't hear the diagnosis, so he looks from me to Jack to Libby to try to ascertain what's being said. I am speechless.

"Do you have any questions?" the doctor asks.

"What's next?" I squeeze out.

"We'll refer you to an oncologist and he'll start you on a protocol as soon as possible. Again, I'm so sorry." We are all silent. "Well, I'll leave you to be with family. I start vacation tomorrow, so if you do have any further questions about the biopsy, you can call my partner. Goodbye."

"Bye," I say, remembering that she told me yesterday she was delaying her trip to Italy so she could do my biopsy. "Have fun in Italy."

The door quietly closes behind her.

One month. One year. Maybe two. No cure. Short straw.

The deafening silence is broken by Jack's sobbing.

And our world comes crashing in.

CHAPTER 6

Ticking time bomb

Jim and Libby have to catch a ferry back to their home on Vashon Island.

Jack and I sit silently in the hospital room. I mean, what do you say? What don't you say? One month. One year. It's like we're in another dimension — a dimension that is completely foreign. I don't feel alive. I don't feel dead. I'm just dangling over some unknown abyss and Jack's on the other side of the abyss. We can see each other, but we're far, far away from one another. We are mute. We are paralyzed. He can't join me, and I can't join him.

I don't want to leave Jack.

"Can you walk me around the unit?" I ask, trying to pull myself out of this … this … place.

"Of course." He moves tubes so I can get out of bed and unplugs the IV stand from the outlet so it can accompany us on our walk. I'm weak and very unstable, so I hold Jack's left arm as I shuffle past other patients' rooms and then past the children's rooms filled with balloons and teddy bears and little people on respirators. We pass an empty room with a stunning view.

"Let's go in here," I say. "Check out the view."

"Gorgeous," he says, looking at the last shadows of a June sunset illuminating Capitol Hill.

Then we fall into each other's arms and start crying.

"I'm going to die," I whisper.

"I know," he says. "I know."

"Go home to Rose," I tell him. "But don't tell her. I want to tell her. And don't tell anyone else. I don't want Rose to be the last to know."

"I don't want to go."

"Go. Be with our daughter," I reiterate. "I'm just going to take a sleeping pill and sleep through the night." He looks at me, tilting his head in doubt. "I'm not going to die tonight!"

"Alright, but …" he sputters.

"I'll. Be. Fine. I promise."

"You're so beautiful. I love you so much. Can I take your picture?"

I nod my head and step back in front of the window with the twinkling city behind me.

He doesn't bother to say, "Smile."

Quite shockingly, I sleep well. I mean, I do take an Ambien after Jack leaves the hospital because I don't want to spend the night looping on my grim diagnosis.

In the morning — shall we call it "the morning after"? — Jack arrives with my favorite breakfast — Chai tea and a savory scone, which I just pick at it because I'm not very hungry. And now of course I know why I'm not hungry, because I have a big fucking tumor in my head pushing on the appetite portion of my thinker.

"You didn't tell anyone, did you?" I ask Jack.

"No," he replies.

"What did you tell Rose?"

"I just told her," he says, pausing, "it wasn't good."

"No, it wasn't good," I agree, trying to be brave. "They said I can check out this morning. We have to make an appointment with that oncologist and turn that month into a year."

"Right," says Jack.

After checking out of the hospital, which seems to take days, we drive the short one and a half miles home. The summer is in full swing. It's sunny. Trees are in bloom and children skip down the sidewalk. The world looks so beautiful.

As we pull in the driveway, I eye the stairs to the front door. There are only seven of them, but that seems like a mountainside to me now.

"Can I take your arm?" I ask, taking Jack's arm.

When we enter the foyer, I call to Rose. She is upstairs. So I climb another mountain of stairs and Rose comes out of her room.

"Hi, Mama," Rose says, standing at her bedroom door. "How are you feeling? Daddy said it didn't go that well."

What am I gonna say to my 16-year-old? How do you tell your child that you won't be there to see her graduate or get married or have babies? There's simply no positive spin you can cast on this news. I try to think of a way to phrase it that will be honest and somehow digestible.

"Baby, I'm dying"? Too blunt.

Maybe soften it with something like, "Sweetie, I love you so much. I will always be here with you, even when I'm not here with you"?

Or, take technical a route? "Honey, I have what's called a medullo-blastoma — it's an inoperable, malignant, fast-growing tumor in my right cerebellum."

One month. One year.

And here she stands before me, asking a glib, almost run-of-the-mill question, "How'd it go?" And now I have to break her heart. I walk into her bedroom and sit on her bed.

"Sit down," I say, patting the mattress next to me.

"Well?" she asks, still in a blissful fog of ignorance.

"Rosie," I say, starting to tear up, "I have an inoperable malignant brain tumor."

Her life of two seconds ago comes to a close. Her childhood ends. Mortality is now part of her existence. I take her in my arms and we both let our emotions pour into each other.

"How long?" she chokes out.

"A month? A year?" I tell her, trying to add the encouraging hope. "Maybe even two years."

I don't want to leave Rose.

The news has cast us into a slow-motion haze. Rose and I tread downstairs and tell our unsuspecting houseguest, Saul. Saul is the 21-year-old son of one of my high school friends, and he's living with us for part of the summer. Having grown up in the English countryside, he's here as a tourist. He's been a welcome presence in our lives, eager to soak up Seattle's beauty, engage in meaningful discussions about growing up in Britain's bucolic Somerset, share his experiences about pursuing an education in Chinese at Cambridge, cook lovely meals for the family, and just provide pleasurable company. Only days ago, we had taken him to the summer solstice parade in the offbeat neighborhood of Fremont to marvel at the naked cyclists and visit our favorite Korean restaurant.

The shock with which he receives the news is apparent, almost embarrassing. This is such an intimate shift in our lives, that it almost feels inappropriate to tell him. But he's living here and keeping a secret like this would be impossible. Besides, why would I? If he's going to remain here during the rest of my short days, he needs to be fully on board with the ensuing challenge. Or leave.

"Would you like me to stay at my aunt's?" he asks me.

"No, Saul," I assure him. "If you can handle the ride, I'd be honored to have you remain with us." Saul feels like family, and the notion of being surrounded by family feels very comforting right now.

"Alright, but if you need your privacy…" he trails off.

"I'll tell you," I promise.

Next on the list is Kathy, my mom. I had assumed I would be her confidant through the end of her life, holding her hand, loving her, laughing with her, and being her best friend through the progression of her Alzheimer's. If I go, she will have few visitors. No one will bring her dog Arthur to see her. She will not get car rides that include

Starbucks visits in front of the gas fireplace. She won't have movie nights with bed snuggles in her room. Her wardrobe and weekly needs will be left up to the staff — and I don't even know if they do that.

Who's going to bring her Reese's Peanut Butter Cups?

I scale the stairs to the first floor, where my mom is doubtless hanging out. I see Janice, the receptionist. She stands to hug me, and I burst into tears.

"What's the matter?" she asks.

"I have terminal brain cancer," I let loose. "I have to tell my mom."

"No!" she exclaims, still hugging me. "Not you! How did this happen?"

"I dunno. I dunno."

One by one, the staff comes forward, hugging me. Kat, the social director looks me in the eye. "You have to stop eating sugar and meat. Are you taking any herbs?" she presses.

"Kat, I just found out," I tell her. "I haven't even started to think about any of that." Out of the corner of my eye, I see my mother sitting in the living room with the other residents.

"I have to tell Kathy," I tell the group.

"Of course! Of course!" they say in unison.

I pull away from the shocked group and walk over to my mother. "Hi, Mom, it's your daughter Deirdre."

"I know who you are," she says. "Where you been, Snot Face?"

"I've been around," I assure her.

"I haven't seen you," she argues.

"I was here a couple of days ago. Wanna sit outside on the deck?" I ask her. "It's beautiful and sunny out. They're serving cookies."

"Yeah," she says, as I help her stand.

We shuffle onto the deck that overlooks Mercer Island and I seat her in a cushioned white wicker settee.

"Here, let me grab you a cookie," I say. I don't know why I'm getting her a cookie. But she loves cookies and somehow it seems like that cookie might comfort her after the blow.

"Thank you, honey," she says, reaching for the confection. "Aren't you gonna have one?"

"Nah, I'm not that hungry," I tell her. "Mom, I have some news for you. It's kinda sad. Do you want to hear it?"

"Yes," she answers.

"OK," I take a deep breath. "I've been diagnosed with terminal brain cancer."

She immediately starts crying. I decide not to show her the shaved spots on my head and my crazy two-inch long set of stitches that are now covered by my hair.

"Why couldn't they take some dumb shit like me?" she cries. "See why I don't believe in God? Oh, my beautiful D-D. And here I thought you were doing so good and looked so thin."

I take my mom to my home for the rest of the day. I want her there as we share the news with family and friends.

The sun is making a rare appearance in our front yard so Jack and Rose start pulling camping chairs into the shifting rays. Jack has started calling close friends who are now heading over, in their own respective states of shock. We've lived in this house for 18 years, so many of our neighbors have become de facto family members. As they walk by, we tell them the news. They walk home and grab more camping chairs and bring wine and snacks. It's a surreal impromptu neighborhood summer party.

It's been two hours since Kathy learned the news. The whole drive to my house, she remembered that I had brain cancer. I was so proud of her for remembering something beyond 10 seconds. But the change in venue, the growing party, the beer she's drinking, the laughing, the crying, have all perked her up and solidly placed her in party mode. Kathy loves a good party.

"My brain's not worth a damn anymore," Kathy says, turning to me.

"It turns out mine isn't either," I joke. I'm beginning to wrap my mind around my new reality. "We're in a race to see whose brain gives out first."

"Why?" she asks.

"Because you have Alzheimer's, and I have brain cancer."

"Who are you?"

"Your daughter."

"Oh, well then that's terrible!"

🍭 🍭 🍭

I've now known about my state for 36 hours. One month. T-Minus 28. I don't know what to do. Do I just stay in bed and die? My bed's very comfortable. Dying people always seem to be in bed on TV or in the movies. But if I live a year, that's a long time to stay in bed just dying. So, I reason, I'll get up. It's Sunday … Jack won't be working. Maybe he'll want to hang out. Then again, Rose is probably still in bed. Maybe I should go die with her for a while in her bed, snuggling. That sounds like a great death.

Then my real alarm goes off … Arthur. As if he receives telepathic communications, every day Arthur starts crying at the bottom of the stairs so I'll get up and take him for a walk — just as I'm waking up. How does he know I'm waking up? I mean, it's not like I wake at the same time every day as people with actual jobs do. And it's not like I wake up to an alarm that Arthur could hear. I just open my eyes and he starts barking. Today, I don't really feel like doing our neighborhood stroll through the woods with our ball-throwing session at Lake Washington.

Jack is downstairs watching TV. "Honey, do you want to you-know-what the d-o-g?" I ask in a half-whisper while spelling out 'dog.' I can't actually say "walk Arthur" because Arthur will start freaking out and barking, "LET'S GO ON A WALK! LET'S GO ON A WALK! LET'S GO ON A WALK!"

"Not really," he says. Jack doesn't like — no, correction — Jack loathes walking Arthur. At 75 pounds, Arthur is a big goofy (read: charmingly untrained) labradoodle who is too big and too rambunctious for Jack's taste. "Have Rose do it."

"Yeah, right," I say. Rose would rather clip a finger off than walk the dog. She'll only walk the dog if someone is dying, which I am, so I'm thinking if I work that angle, I might be able to wiggle out of my doggy duties today.

I gingerly go upstairs to see if I can sell Rose on walking the dog. I tap quietly on her door and walk in.

"Rose," I start. "Do you wanna walk Arthur?"

"Ohhh," she rolls over, smelling like candy and sleep. "Noooo, Mama."

"Please? We can walk together," I say, like that'll make it fun.

"I just don't want to. Is it OK if I just don't?" she asks. "Maybe Daddy can?"

Sometimes, this family, I think in exasperation. *I'm dying everyone. Walk the dog for me*!

But somehow, even my imminent demise doesn't shake my family into wanting to assume that chore. I am the dog walker. Period.

"OK honey," I concede, silently pissed. But for whatever reason, I want to maintain in Rose's mind that things are business as usual. "Sleep well. Sorry to bother you."

I go back downstairs and open 'the drawer.' It's the doggie drawer that contains combs and brushes and leashes and collars. Arthur hears 'the drawer' open and goes ballistic.

"WE'RE GOING ON THE WALK! WE'RE GOING ON THE WALK! WE'RE GOING ON THE WALK!" He barks his deafening bark while jumping on me.

"Arthur! Get down!" I admonish. He keeps jumping on me.

As we head down the street, it's like a scene out of "The Truman Show." I literally run into EVERY neighbor I know as Arthur pulls me down the sidewalk.

"Hey," says my next-door-neighbor. "How you doin'?"

This is one of the neighbors who didn't pow wow with us last night. I do believe we can get too rambunctious (drunk) with our friends (also drunk) for their liking on the occasional Friday night.

"I'm OK," I say, so accustomed am I to that rejoinder. "But did you hear I've been diagnosed with terminal brain cancer?"

"I did hear," she replies. "I'm sorry. My dad died of cancer."

"Yeah," I say. "I'm sorry."

"Thanks," she says. "How you feelin'?"

"Um, OK, except for the news that I'm dying," I say. "And my dizziness is driving me crazy."

"What's it like?" she asks.

"It's not room-spinning dizziness," I explain. "It's more like I'm drunk on a boat."

"Yeah, my dad had lung cancer," she repeats. "But he smoked all of his life, so …"

"Yeah, that can happen with smoking," I say, turning to Arthur pulling on the leash. "OK, well I have to help this beast run off some of his energy. See ya later."

"See ya," she says. "And, I'm sorry to hear your news."

"Yeah, me too," I nod.

As I walk away, I think, *That went well. I didn't crack a single tear. I can do this.*

The next neighbor I run into I met when our daughters started kindergarten together. She's a Christian Scientist with an old-world penchant for sending me the occasional letter of encouragement in the mail. Not on Facebook. Not in a text. Not on Twitter. But a real genuine letter on real genuine paper with a real genuine Forever Stamp.

"Deirdre," she waves from across the street. "How are you?"

I cross the street and look at her. "Oh Anne," I start hugging her and crying, unable to hold back the news. "I've been diagnosed with terminal brain cancer."

"Deirdre, I'm so sorry," she comforts me. The comforting moment passes quickly as Arthur pulls, barking, "LET'S GET TO THE BEACH, MOM! GET TO THE BEACH! BEACH!"

"Clearly Arthur's not concerned," I sniffle. "I better go. Sorry I lost it on you."

"If there is anything I can do — anything — I'm right here," she says, holding my hand.

"Thank you, Anne," I say. "I will let you know."

As I walk away, I start thinking, What will I need? What do dying people need? I used to volunteer at hospice doing caregiver relief. Four hours a week I would clean, cook, watch movies, read out loud — do whatever the patient desired while I was there. Usually, they just wanted a neutral person to speak to and a friend to watch Friends with.

I start to make a mental list of things I might need help with:

1) The dogs. Specifically, the dogwalking. Well, you know how that sells around my house.

2) Cleaning the house. Based on the past 25 years, I haven't ever seen any of my family display the ability (or desire) to clean, so that may have to be outsourced.

3) Loading (and running, and emptying) the dishwasher. I will have to coach my housemates that putting dishes in the dirty sink does not constitute 'doing the dishes.'

4) Doing the laundry. Again, I will have to coach my house-mates that 'doing the laundry' does not mean throwing their dirties down the laundry chute. It actually involves throwing the laundry down the chute, dividing it into colors and whites, putting it in the washer (with detergent), setting the washer on start, moving the now-clean laundry from the washer to the dryer (with a softener), transferring it from the dryer to an empty laundry basket when it's dry, folding it, and then, putting all of the now-clean laundry AWAY. That may have to be outsourced too. Maybe Anne can do that. She did offer "anything."

5) Gardening. I'm no gardener, but my yard doth get thirsty in the summer and she doth love to host a proliferating population of dandelions and blackberry bushes. She will go feral if someone doesn't do a modicum of nature control.

6) Taking care of my mother.

And then I stop.

Where am I going? Where is she going? As dedicated atheists, my parents raised us to believe there is no heaven or hell or god or after-life. Life. Just. Ends. What does "end" mean? Will it be like entering a black hole with nothingness, abso-fucking-lutely nothingness? Will there be angels and harps or (gasp) fork-tongued devils in fiery pits? For the first time in my life, I don't want to be an atheist. I like the idea of entering some infinite divine where my soul will convene with the wisdom of the universe and I will be able to make 'trips' home to watch over my loved ones. I commit to spend the next few weeks talking to anyone and everyone about their beliefs on the hereafter. Maybe, just maybe, I'll be able to come to some comfortable accep-tance that even though my physical life will be shutting down, my spiritual existence will soar.

Then my thoughts turn back to Kathy. Who will take care of my mother? As I begin to cycle on this worry, I realize that this is going to be one of my biggest challenges: setting up my world so it can run smoothly without me. I'll need to figure out some sort of schedule so my mom has regular visitors to bring joy to her confused loneliness. Somebody to sit with her who knew her when. Somebody who can put a smile on her face with her kind of humor. Somebody to bring her a Reese's.

What about Rose? I'm about to leave my baby girl motherless. Will she have a nervous breakdown and flunk out of school? Will she start using drugs to 'kill the pain'? Will Jack remarry, and will Rose love her new mom? Will her new mom look like me? Will she be young? More importantly, will she be younger than me? Will she be naturally thin and athletic? Why haven't I been more thin and athletic? Will she be funny? I'm funny … but will she be funnier than me? Will she rock Jack's world in bed? Why haven't I been a better lover for him? Will he love Rose's new mom more than he loved me? Will Rose have this new mom in her wedding photos and at her baby's first birth? Will Rosemary's mother-in-law step in and love her like a daughter and help care for her children? How long before they all start forgetting what my voice sounded like and how much I loved my morning tea and my long walks with the dogs and how I cackled unabashedly watching "America's Funniest Home Videos"? When will they finally disable my Facebook, Tumblr and email accounts?

How long before I become a dusty memory?

When Arthur and I return from our two-mile jaunt, Sue is sitting in the living room with Jack. Like Anne, Sue came into our world when our children started kindergarten at the same school. Her son, Hadley, became one of Rose's closest friends over the years, starting with messy playdates at 5, and developing into a dedicated friendship that carries on today.

Sue stands and comes over to me with a firm sisterly hug.

"Deirdre, I hope you don't mind," she says, sitting down next to me. "I've taken the liberty of reading up on your cancer." Sue is a former nurse and now a therapist. Her husband, Al, is an ear, nose and throat doctor. "I've perused these two books by progressive doctors, David Servan-Schreiber's "Anti Cancer" (Viking Penguin, 2009) and Keith Block's "Life Over Cancer" (Bantam Dell, 2009). Right now, they're considered some of the primary sources for patients undergoing cancer treatment. They offer innovative approaches from diet and supplements to lifestyle and integrative treatments."

"OK," I say. But really I'm thinking, *this is terminal. I have a month to a year. Why bother reading anything?*

"I've highlighted sections that may be beneficial as you go through treatment," she continues, leafing through a thick book with yellow highlights, pink highlights, notes written in the margins, and Post-it notes sticking out from various pages. My head starts to spin. "What you're about to go through is very traumatic and there can be long-term damage."

"Like death?" I ask, half-jokingly.

"Well, the idea is that treatment will kill the tumor," she continues. "But the treatment itself is so damaging, it would be great if you could focus on surviving the treatment as intact as possible. It is vital that you start preparing your body for the beating it's about to take. These books contain specific diets for various cancers — including brain cancer. There are inspirational stories of success and what worked for other patients. There are explanations of different treatments and their effects. But most importantly, these books will show you how to prepare yourself so that you survive this in the most non-damaging way."

"Thank you, Sue," I say. "Thank you so much."

"There's an integrative doctor in Canada who is on the leading edge of Eastern and Western treatment. We are friends with him and I'd be happy to call him to see if he can see you and give you a treatment plan outside of what your oncologists prescribe. He'll be able to tell you what herbs and alternative treatments may help … All of this would be in addition to whatever Western treatment you receive. I'm telling you, it's not just going to help you survive this, but it will help you survive this well, so you can go back to your life and be fully functional."

"I would like that," I say, thinking my attention is waning and I want to sleep. "Maybe you can give this to Jack?"

"Oh, yes, we've already been talking about it," she says. "He's going to read the books and help you."

"Good," I say. "Because frankly, I don't know if I'm up to reading all this right now."

"I understand," she sympathizes. "I'll keep doing research too, and if Al and I can help in any way, let me know."

"I will," I promise. "Thank you, Sue."

"OK, I'll leave you to rest. But please, before treatment even starts, get a jump-start on your alternative care so you're as strong as possible when the Western treatment begins. It could make all the difference in the world."

I've never been one for 'alternative care.' As a nurse trained in the '50s, my mom always pooh-poohed mumbo-jumbo medical practices like meditation and massage and acupuncture.

"That's all bullshit!" she would emphatically claim. She was so sure of herself that I was confident in turning my nose up at anything that didn't smack of white coats, sterile institutions and over-flowing pill bottles … until now.

While Sue's barrage of thoughts and advice confuse and scare me, I'm happy she's thinking in terms of survival and life after treatment. The game has changed, and I realize that all of my former sarcastic doubt about things I can't see or understand no longer serve me. I have to grab every thread of help, even if the results are unknown. Now, I want to round up all the help I can get … even if it involves incantations, hairy armpits, meditations and patchouli.

I'm a new kind of celebrity — the 'dying person.'

Tonight we're joining Lisa and Andrew — again — friendships made via Rosemary's friends. They're hosting a small dinner party with us and some other friends.

With my newfound celebrity, people freely hug me, tear up, offer me their seats, and look deeply into my eyes as they ask how I'm feeling. My common rejoinder has become, "I'm not in any pain, just dizzy and tired." And that's the truth … I'm in no actual pain. I'm just tired and dizzy.

Then I notice Mary. She's sitting across the room, NOT looking at me or talking to me. Hmm, that's odd, I think. Why won't Mary look at me? Then, I realize, she's frightened to look at me. I am death. And death is frightening.

"Mary," I say. "It's OK. You can look at me. I'm still here."

Mary dabs her eyes. "I just don't know what to say," she admits.

"It's OK," I tell her, "I don't know what to say either. But know that I'm not sad or in any pain."

"How can you not be sad?" she asks.

Well there's a question. Why aren't I sad? I'm crying a lot, but it's like I'm opening myself to the reckoning of an end. My end. And what brings me to tears is feeling the love of those around me and knowing that this love will soon fizzle. And I always return to Rose and my mother and the loss I feel for leaving them. Jack too, but I know he'll be able to find another wife. He's young and handsome. After a mourning period, he can have love again. But Rose can never have another mom. And Kathy can never have another daughter.

And then I realize, I am sad. I'm sadder than fuck. But I don't want to let sadness drive what's ahead of me, and for now, I'm trying to lean my weight against the door to sadness.

Sitting on Andrew and Lisa's deck sipping wine, I look out over Lake Washington. Conversation is quiet among my usually verbose friends. Mary continues to steal glances of me and dab her eyes. But I feel removed from the scene. It is like I am sitting on the precipice of an endless dark canyon containing the vast unknown. Looking out at the blue sky, I feel my soul slowly departing this physical plane and floating up into the heavens as I step ever closer to the canyon's precipice. Visually, it's like my soul is a big piece of chewing gum or Silly Putty, and it's being stretched out of me and pulled upwards.

Oh my God, I think, my soul is leaving and I soon shall follow.

It's been four days since diagnosis. T-Minus 26. There are a few personal things I want to tend to.

I sift through my closets and drawers, throwing away my old stained underwear, my holey socks, my clothes that never fit right, my misguided Goodwill purchases. I don't want Rose to have to troll through my embarrassing intimates and see how disorganized my drawers are or what poor taste I have.

I empty almost 20 years of email from my Hotmail account — the only email account I've ever really had. Ditto my Facebook messages. I think about deleting all of my online accounts, but then I decide to wait until I'm closer to the end.

I make a list of all my accounts — Hotmail, YouTube, Facebook, Tumblr, online banking — with all the passwords, just in case I die before I can shut them down. This way Jack can close them for me.

I start to write my own obit. My first real job was at a newspaper writing obits, and I've become our family's obit writer. Who better than me to get the dates right, remember to include all the pertinent survivors, and slip a joke or two into my final biography?

I file my living will that instructs medical institutions not to resuscitate me or put me on life support once I become a vegetable. I even think of going to my doctor to secure a prescription for an end-of-life concoction just in case I'm in a lot of pain and I want to end it.

And I ponder. I ponder THE END, taking great comfort in the fact that I have accomplished as much as I need to in this life. I have lived every day as I've wanted. I've chased dreams. I've traveled the world — teaching English in Japan, living in Brussels where Jack attended graduate school, touring through much of China and Europe with Jack and Rose. I've made movies and seen life through others' eyes while working as a reporter and a documentarian. I've built great friendships. I've loved and been loved. I have no regrets.

While my time bomb ticks down, my soulful levity intensifies as my previously unacknowledged soul peacefully stretches upward. Though I still sense that I am teetering on the ledge of an ominous dark canyon, the feeling of evaporating from this world and serenely moving into the next, undefined existence, intensifies.

With what little time I have left, I decide that I want my final days to be as good as my life has been.

♀ ♀ ♀

We are now five days into my diagnosis.

As Jack's passion for smoking meats grows, he has created monthly brisket raves called Seattle Brisket Experience (SBX). SBX works like this: Jack books a location such as a distillery or a brewery, he smokes brisket, sausage and chicken, my friend Abby and I prepare the side dishes, and we rope friends into helping us serve food and bartend. The sell-out events have garnered Jack a huge fan club, many of whom are getting increasingly irked because reservations get nabbed up within minutes of Jack announcing the next meat party, and getting a seat at a table has become near unto impossible. Our next is to be hosted on July Fourth at our friends' Chinese restaurant, Chungee's, on Capitol Hill.

"I have to cancel SBX," he tells me. "It's just so wrong for me to cook and entertain when you're …" he couldn't finish the sentence. "I have to quit it all and take care of you."

"No," I tell him. "If I die, this may be the last time I see some of these people. Plus, you'll need something to occupy your time when I'm gone. And if I don't die, then you will have a whole new dream — your restaurant — to chase with me. Either way, you have to carry on. You have to smoke. The future Jack's BBQ is in the balance!"

That night, some dear friends drop by for dinner. As we sit with them, we plot Jack's next SBX. They'll help carry the meats and side dishes to the location. We'll delegate another group to decorate the location. Because I'm now so weak, Abby will manage the kitchen team to make the sides.

Abby and I met 25 years ago when our husbands were both graduate students at Boston University's Brussels branch. As the only wives who had followed our husbands to Europe for schooling, we immediately forged a friendship commiserating on the impossible employment situation for post-college Americans (well, she's Canadian, same difference but with a few "eh?"s tacked on) and the bizarre loneliness of being in a strange country with AWOL husbands who are working on internships during the days and attending classes during the evenings. Our friendship waned after Jack and I moved back to Seattle and she and her husband moved to London and we both started careers and families. They later moved to New Jersey for his career. Unfortunately, Abby''s husband died tragically during a meeting at Windows on the World at the top of the World Trade Center building on 9/11. To escape the many debilitating reminders of her husband's tragic passing, Abby loaded up her two young children and moved to Seattle. And ever since, we've been true-blue BFFs.

Nobody but Abby has the balls to mention my situation. In fact, I find it odd that nobody even asks me about it unless I bring it up.

While it feels callous, I recognize that this silence is becoming a pattern of denial — when you face something so extreme, it pushes all sorts of buttons in people that probably have nothing to do with you. Your dying stirs up traumatic memories of other lost loves or painful experiences that they've had. Or they're just embarrassed to acknowledge the elephant in the room.

"You can't stop now. Now is when you need your passion to distract you," Abby tells Jack without elucidating why he would need a distraction. "I'll get some volunteers to make the sides and recruit a team of servers. Deirdre won't have to worry about a thing."

I don't know if it's because she's experienced deep loss with the death of her husband or if she's always been so damn practical, but she's making sense and we know it.

On the day of SBX our friends come to the house to help make the sides — remoulade coleslaw and Texas caviar. While chopping vegetables, shredding cabbage and opening cans, they lightly banter about their kids and their daily lives in the kitchen. Meanwhile, I swaddle on the couch in the nearby living room, wrapped in blankets and listening to the white noise of conviviality. Every so often, somebody checks on me with sympathetic smiles and tastings of what they're preparing.

As they start loading the prepared meats and sides, I rise from my wraps and take a shower, bracing myself on the tile wall so I don't fall.

The party is a success. The food is good. The music is beautiful. The guests are pleased. Jack assumes his role as the charismatic host. Fireworks illuminate the sky in the distance. At this moment on this warm evening, it seems there could be no finer place to be.

For three whole hours, nobody mentions cancer.

ⓞ ⓞ ⓞ

It's now seven days after receiving my diagnosis. T-Minus 23. Today, I will visit the oncologist my brain surgeon referred me to.

I feel incredibly light. It's partly physical; I now only weigh 123 pounds at 5 feet 11 inches. It's partly mental; I just can't remember much, and I've quit trying. And it's partly soulful; my soul putty continues to stretch toward the heavens as my connection to this world becomes more and more tenuous.

I check in with the receptionist and I can tell I'm developing a fey look in my eyes — sort of seeing through people as I speak to them. It's as if I'm half here.

I've become mentally compromised (really stupid). I'm assuming it's because there's a brain growing inside my brain and this blossoming embryonic cell growth is pushing significantly on the part of my thinker that helps me receive information, understand it, remember it and act on it. Because of this, I've brought a posse of clear thinkers with me to hear what the doctor says: my brother, Don, who has a background in science; my niece, Kimmie, who has been rocked to her core by my diagnosis; and Jack, who ultimately will have to hold my hand through every moment of my treatment.

"Deirdre?" calls out the nurse.

"Yes, here," I say, standing.

"Follow me," she instructs. "We'll be in Room 3."

We all stand and walk silently to my room. While Jack and Don have been doing a lot of reading about my situation since this began, I haven't. Every time I start to read about brain cancer I get sick to my stomach and just want to crawl into a hole and get it all over with. So, I've just shut out researching anything about my situation and instead tried to enjoy every single moment.

After the nurse takes my vitals, she announces Dr. G will be in soon.

An affable blue-eyed man in a white lab coat enters.

"Hello, I'm Dr. G," he announces. "And who's my patient?" he asks, looking at the four of us.

"I am," I say, standing and extending my hand. "Hi, I'm Deirdre."

"Deirdre! How are you?" he asks, somewhat rhetorically.

"Well, I'm dying of cancer," I say.

"Balderdash!" he exclaims. "Let's look at the facts. You have a medulloblastoma. You know that already."

"Yes," I answer.

"Now, this is a curious thing. You have a tumor that normally affects children — actually, babies. It is leftover embryonic cells that usually die after birth, but sometimes they live on and lay dormant. How old are you?"

"Forty-seven," I tell him.

"Right," he says, looking at my chart. "That's what's so puzzling. Medulloblastomas are common in children, but very rare in adults, and almost unheard of in someone past 20. That's why the radiologists had such a difficult time diagnosing it."

"How did I get it?" I ask.

"That's the million-dollar question," he says. "When your immune system is compromised, these cells are opportunists and start reproducing. But they almost never survive long enough after birth to become a concern. Let me ask you this: How do you think you got it?"

Reflecting on the past four years, I get tired just thinking about all the balls I've been juggling: Parents, daughter, work, pets, marriage, life.

"I don't know," I answer. "The past couple of years have been stressful. Maybe my immune system was compromised?"

I've been drinking Tab and Diet Coke since I was 9 years old. My dad would always look at me disapprovingly as I downed each soda. "Those are filled with neurotoxins."

"Diet soda?" I ask the doctor. "My dad always said it had neuro-toxins."

In 1977 when I was 12, my parents moved us from Kansas to Seattle. Our newly constructed home boasted a magical new gadget — a microwave. My parents were so worried about the microwave, they made us turn it on and run out of the kitchen so we didn't get brain cancer from any radioactive waves that might escape the solid glass door.

"Maybe microwaves?" I guess.

Jack bought me an early generation cell phone — the big kind with an antenna. So taken with my novel toy, I used it constantly, amazing my friends that I could call them while driving or shopping or hitting the beach. But that phone, boy, it would heat up the right side of my brain. "Well, I better hang up," I remember saying with most every call. "My phone is cooking my brain."

"Cell phones?" I guess again.

On one of my preposterous diets I injected human chorionic go-nadotropin into my belly for a month and only ate 500 calories a day. Hcg is a hormone produced during pregnancy — maybe it woke up my embryonic cells and produced a tumor? But this potential cause is just too embarrassing to list, so I say nothing.

Then my mind wanders to Hanford, and processed foods, and plastics, and airport X-rays, and genetically modified foods, and my proclivity to drink, and American-style inactivity of too much TV and too little exercise and then I think, *how could I NOT have cancer???*

"You had steroid injections in your neck at one time, am I cor-rect?" Dr. G asks.

"Yes, about five years ago," I answer. I had a herniated disk in my neck that caused tremendous pain as it pushed against my spinal cord, making my left shoulder and arm feel as if they'd been shot with a rifle.

"I'm suspicious of those," he says. "But let's talk about the future, because that's what matters now, right?"

"My future? We know it ain't pretty," I say.

The doctor seems so upbeat, which seems rude, what with my dying and all. I guess he's just used to dying cancer patients.

"Not necessarily!" he tells me. "There is a 60 percent chance of success in treating medulloblastomas in adults. With chemo and radiation, we can rat out this beast. And there are also some new clinical trials that are genome-mapping brain cancer and they're even more promising."

And then, the strangest thing happens. There is almost a visceral snap as I feel my soul fly back from the heavens and join me here on Earth. Sixty percent chance? Those are odds I can work with.

Jack, Kimmie and Don collectively look at each other as if thinking, "Game on!"

"So, what next?" I ask, trying to hold back tears of relief and joy.

"I'd like to do a lumbar puncture," he continues. "Medulloblastomas like to travel to the spine. So before we do anything else, we need to see if it's traveled. I'd also like to send a sample of your biopsy to the lab and see what kind of medullo we're dealing with. That can also impact your chances of survival. Do you approve of us sending in a sample?"

"Yes! Yes! Whatever it takes!" I exclaim.

"And the lumbar puncture?"

"Puncture away!" I bubble.

"Are you free tomorrow?" he asks.

"Yes, I'm free tomorrow," I say. "What time? Any time."

"Alright," the doctor concludes. "I'll have the nurse book you for the puncture tomorrow and I'll see you then."

As he stands to leave, I hug him. This man has just imbued me with hope that I may survive.

After we leave the doctor's office, Jack, Don, Kimmie and I hug and cry. I dance out to the parking lot, looking like Elaine on "Seinfeld" with her bad dancing because I'm now so uncoordinated. Driving home, Jack and I are like giddy children.

"Woot woot!" I shout out. "Can you believe that fucking surgeon telling me there was NO cure???" I exclaim, riding high on the news that I stand a chance. "I mean, a 60 percent chance of survival? Why the hell was she even calling out my prognosis? All she had to say was, 'You have a malignant brain tumor called a medulloblastoma in your right cerebellum. I'll refer you to an oncologist, and he'll discuss treatment from here.'"

"I know," says Jack, beaming.

"I'm gonna li-ive, I'm gonna li-ive," I start singing.

I pull out my cellphone and call Rose. I've kept her away from doctor's appointments and all of the various testing because I don't want hospital beds and needles and painful truths to be her final memories of me. I've wanted to shield her from this ugly reality and reserve our time together in the cozy home she grew up in enjoying what little time we have left. But now … I'm calling my baby with the news of what feels like my own rebirth.

"I'm going to live!" I tell her. "Nana-a-boo-boo, I'm gonna li-ive!"

"Oh Mama," is all she says, crying into the phone.

When I get home, I call my friend Abby.

"Congratulations!" Abby says. "How are we going to celebrate your life?"

"Now don't get jealous, but I will be celebrating the big news with a lumbar puncture tomorrow," I say.

"Do you want me to come with you?" she offers.

"No das OK," I say, still just so happy that I have a fighting chance. "My niece Kimmie, my brother Don and Jack are coming along. But I'll call you after the lumbar puncture and we can celebrate."

As we enter the doctor's office the next day, I am keenly aware that my vision is no longer unfocused. I am here and completely present without the sense that I am straddling two dimensions.

"Deirdre?" the receptionist asks.

"*C'est moi,*" I sing.

"Come on in," she directs, handing me a hospital gown. "You'll need to disrobe and wear these."

Don and Jack stay in the waiting room because for Don it's awkward being present at an intimate (read: naked body) procedure, and Jack is goobered out by watching things like tubes puncturing spines. Kimmie and I settle into my room, I don the now-familiar-patterned hospital gown while Kimmie ties the straps at the back of my neck.

Dr. G enters and has me crawl on the exam table and assume a fetal position.

"You're going to have to go into a really tight curl," the nurse tells me, then turns to Kimmie. "Can you push her head down while I push her legs tight into her chest?"

The two women put their weight against me, holding me in a tight curl.

"You OK Deirdre?" the doctor asks.

"Yeah."

"OK, Little prick where I'm injecting the anesthesia … feel that?" he asks.

"Oh yes. Ow! OK. I feel that."

After letting that sit for a second, the doctor turns his attention to Kimmie.

You'll need to press on Deirdre more firmly now," he says. "The idea is we open up the spinal cord as much as possible."

"OK," she says.

Between Kimmie and the nurse, I feel like I'm being compressed to the size of a volleyball.

"First we'll inject a local anesthetic," the doctor says, pricking the middle of my neck and injecting some painkiller. He rubs the area of the injection for a few seconds. "Can you feel that?"

"Yes," I say. "No, wait. No. It's going numb," I report.

"OK, good. Ladies, make sure you're pushing her as tightly as you can," he instructs. I feel like they're making me tiny enough to slide right back into my mother's womb and I silently thank the years of yoga that have made my body pliable enough to withstand this mini-torture. "Deirdre, you'll feel a little bit of pressure here."

I feel the pressure and try to distract myself from the fact that a tube is going into my spine by envisioning puppies and kittens.

"And we're in," he says. "How you doin'?"

"Fine," I squeeze out. Then I think how awkward and yet how funny it would be if I farted right at this moment. I start to laugh.

"Everything OK?" asks the doctor.

"Yeah, yeah, sorry." I figure I don't need to explain myself. It would be distracting and all, which may not be cool with a tube stuck in my spine.

"OK," says the doctor as I feel the pressure ease. "Ladies, you can quit compressing Deirdre." Then to me, "This is a good sign."

I roll over on my back to see Dr. G holding up a vial of what looks like holy water.

"It's clear," he points out. "If it's discolored or cloudy, that can be a sign of infection, or worse…"

"So, the tumor hasn't traveled to my spine?" I ask.

"That we can't decipher with the human eye. We'll have to send this to the lab for testing," he explains. "We'll know by tomorrow if the tumor has spread."

"And if it has?" I ask.

"That's not good," is all he says.

I put my clothes on. My hubris at having a 60 percent chance of survival is suddenly deflated by this new risk. What if … what if it's beyond brain cancer?

The next day, it is with equal parts fear and excitement that I return to Dr. G's office. Jack and Don have joined me again since I know they're going to tell me things I need to understand, and more importantly, remember.

As we're whisked toward the exam room, Dr. G meets us in the hall and follows us in.

"I have exciting news," he says.

Just his tone tells me the tumor hasn't sent out satellite cells to my spine.

"Your spine is clean, no cancer," he says.

"Oh, that is great," says Don.

"But there's something else," Dr. G continues. "Here, look at this," he says, sitting down at a computer.

He enters a government database that lists worldwide clinical trials for various ailments. He scrolls down to one listed for medulloblastomas.

"Now, from your brain sample, the lab has determined that you have what's called a Sonic Hedgehog," he says. "It's a very specific kind of medulloblastoma, and it just so happens that they're conducting genome-mapping trials with Sonic Hedgehog medullos. The trial is in Phase 3, which means they're past the testing phase and now trying to get it approved for market. Now get this: With relapse patients, the trial has a 70 percent success rate."

"Is it experimental?" I ask.

"Yes, but the results are very promising," he says.

"What about traditional treatment?" Jack asks. "They have a pretty high success rate."

"Well, yes. But with these new genome-mapping treatments you get to avoid the toxic effects of chemo and radiation."

But, I'm thinking, *the traditional treatment of chemo and radiation is a well-traveled road and the success rates are high. I don't necessarily want to be a guinea pig on some clinical trial. No sirree, not today.*

"And even more interesting is UW is one of the hospitals participating in the trial, so you wouldn't even need to travel."

"OK, but how would you treat this if I don't go the route of clinical trials?" I ask.

"Well, there's a weekly brain conference tomorrow and I will consult with other doctors who specialize in brain cancer to design a traditional treatment," he explains.

"Have you ever … treated a medulloblastoma?" I ask.

"No, but I'm excited at the prospect," he answers honestly.

And all of a sudden, I feel like some high-school geek's fascinating science fair project.

When Jack and I get home, Jack calls our friend and doctor Al and shares his reservations about the oncologist we've been referred to.

"There are basically two teams who excel at treating brain cancer in Seattle," Al tells Jack. "It would be advisable to meet them, if just to get second and third opinions. If you like, I can introduce you to one of teams at University of Washington Medical Center."

"Would you?" I ask. "I think I'd like that. I mean, I love my current doctor, but he's never treated a medullo …"

"I understand," says Al. "It's always best to research the specialists and at least talk to them. You want to be as informed as possible as you go into treatment, and the doctors at UW work with Seattle

Children's Hospital, who work with a lot of medulloblastomas in children."

The next day, Jack and Don and Kimmie I head to the Neurology Clinic at UW, an expansive hangar-like structure with a three-story window overlooking a small stand of trees in a grassy field. It's impressive in its aesthetic.

After filling out the tedious forms chronicling my medical history for the umpteenth time, the nurse calls us in to meet UW's brain tumor rock stars comprised of a chemo oncologist, a surgeon and a radiation oncologist. Our first visit is with the brain surgeon.

"As you know," he says, "Your tumor is inoperable, so there's no role for me in your treatment."

Unlike a free-floating tumor that can be surgically removed (think of a cherry or a plum sitting in your brain), my tumor is interstitial and growing throughout the right cerebellum (think of the roots of a tree spreading underground). In order to remove my tumor surgically, they would have to remove my right cerebellum — and we don't want that. I like that cerebellum. I need that cerebellum. It's what regulates my motor movement, balance, coordination, posture and speech.

Because my right cerebellum is swelling like a Fukushima cabbage and pushing on my brain, I can't walk a straight line, let alone tango or tap dance. My ability to write by hand or even type is becoming very, very, very challenging. More often than not, I now ask one of my medical escorts to complete my lengthy forms. I quit driving after Dr. G rightly advised me to stay away from the steering wheel. Yesterday on a short hike with Saul and Rose through the woods in my neighborhood, I simply fell off the path and into a bush.

Since the surgeon has no use for me and my inoperable friend, he kicks me to the chemo oncologist.

In walks a blue-eyed physician: he's wearing a suit; he's svelte; he's groomed within an inch of his life.

"As you know," Dr. G starts, "it's very rare to have a medulloblastoma at your age. In fact, you're somewhat of an international celebrity — brain tumor specialists worldwide know about your brain."

I think of Mary Katherine Gallagher on "Saturday Night Live." I kinda want to stuff my fingers into my armpits and jump up yelling "Super Starrrr!" But I just nod my head.

"I've been in contact with Children's Hospital to see if their medullo specialist wants to take you on," he says. "Unfortunately, you're too old. They simply don't handle patients over 18."

*Ageist*s, I think.

"But we will be in constant contact with them as we create your protocol," he says.

"What's a protocol?" I ask.

"Your treatment plan?" he responds as if I should've known that term.

"Oh, my protocol," I stress, as if maybe I just misheard him. In truth, I had no idea a treatment plan was called a protocol.

"What are we looking at?" Jack thankfully interjects. *God, don't let me talk to these people*, I think, *I don't even know the word for 'treatment.'*

"Inoperable medulloblastomas are typically treated in two stages, the first being six weeks of aggressive radiation on your brain and down your spine coupled with a powerful chemo push once a week."

"What's a push?" I ask.

"Basically, a 15-minute infusion of chemo," he explains.

"And then she's finished?" Jack asks.

"No. That's just the first stage of treatment," he continues. "When that's complete, we'll follow up with nine rounds of chemo, which I doubt Deirdre will be able to finish. Kids can tolerate chemo much better than adults and at 47, Deirdre will probably only be able to handle five or six sessions of chemo infusions, but we'll push it until her blood is no longer recuperating quickly enough."

"Ever?" I ask.

"No, just during the course of treatment. Ultimately your blood will rebound."

"Have you ever treated a medulloblastoma?" Jack asks.

"Yes, a few," Dr. C responds.

"How did they ... do?" Jack asks.

"They're all still alive," the doctor confidently says.

"We've heard there's a highly-successful clinical trial going that treats the kind of medulloblastoma Deirdre has," Jack throws out. "What about getting her into that trial?"

"That's only for relapse patients that have already been through radiation," he says. "Deirdre doesn't qualify."

"Well, is chemo and radiation her only choice?" he presses on.

"If she wants to live," he says.

I'm still not used to someone discussing my eminent future in terms of life and death. As Dr. C stands and shakes everyone's hands,

I start to slide back into what I'm beginning to identify as "the sixth dimension." In this room of people, I'm not really like them anymore. They're solidly alive and vibrant while my future balances over a dark void. Feeling positive just minutes ago, now I feel like I'm re-entering a game of Manhunt without a controller or a weapon.

The radiation oncologist — the third leg of the tumor team — enters, shadowed by three kids.

"Hi," she shakes my hand efficiently. "I'm Dr. H. Do you mind if some of our resident doctors are present during this meeting?"

"No, by all means," I say. Actually, their presence irritates me. I can barely handle today's data dump and this unexpected audience irks me. Plus, they're SO YOUNG it's almost insulting. How can they appreciate a mother struggling for her life? Shouldn't they be out riding tricycles or licking rainbow lollipops? "We all have to learn."

"Great," Dr. H clips. "So, scanning your MRIs, we're looking at a fairly aggressive radiation plan," she begins. "I work with proton therapy. The advantage of proton therapy over photon therapy …"

"I'm sorry, what?" Shit, I can't keep track of all this. "Are you guys following this?" I turn to Don and Jack.

"Yeah," they both answer. Show-offs.

"Photon therapy and proton therapy are different forms of radiation," the doctor slows down for the dummy in the crowd. "With photon therapy, we shoot photons at the tumor. The only problem with that is the photons are like a bullet: They enter one side and exit out the other side, which means any organs on the other side of where you're being treated will also be radiated causing a lot of collateral damage. In your case, that's not good — we'll be radiating your brain and your whole spine, meaning every major organ could be damaged by photon exit rays."

"Wait, why are you radiating my spine? It hasn't traveled to my spine," I point out.

"As a precautionary measure. medullos like to travel to the spine and that test was more than a week ago," she explains. "You have a Grade 4 tumor, which means it's fast-growing. We can't take any chances."

"What about proton therapy?" asks Jack.

"Right, so with proton therapy the protons are extracted with a nuclear accelerator. When the protons hit the tumor, they die on contact without exiting out the other side. It's like a grenade versus a bullet — protons stop on impact whereas photons keep traveling, causing that collateral damage."

"Is proton therapy ... safe?" I ask.

"The goal is to kill very specific cells in your brain," she says, skirting the question. "That's our science, treating the tumor without killing you. And we're very good at it."

"Oh, good," I say. *Oh God*, I think.

"You need to be aware of the potential long-term damage," she continues at rapid fire. She's standing up. I wish everyone would leave and she would just sit down, take my hand, and speak to me at eye level. She raises her machine gun and continues her barrage. "Radiation can damage your thyroid, and lifelong hypothyroidism is not an unusual result."

"For the rest of my life?" I ask. I think hypothyroidism makes you fat.

"Yes, but it's alright," she assures me. "Hypothyroidism is easily treated with a daily medication."

"Yay," I say.

"Your heart and lungs can also be impacted as well as your hearing and vision," she shoots. "You will lose your short-term memory."

"Completely?" I ask.

"Probably," she says.

None of this is what I want to hear.

"Is my hair going to fall out?"

"Well, yes," she answers, as if that's obvious.

"But it will grow back, right?" I ask. I mean, I assumed it would fall out. Being bald is signature cancer style. It's what differentiates us from the rest of the pack.

"No, it will never grow back," she says.

"What? Never?" I don't believe this.

"No, never," she reiterates.

"What about my facial hair, like the hair on my chin and upper lip?" I ask.

"I don't know about that, but you can expect your eyelashes and eyebrows to fall out," she breezes.

"Wait, will my eyelashes and eyebrows grow back?" I ask, sliding into a very frightening vision of post-treatment Deirdre.

"I can't guarantee it."

"Will I lose weight?"

"Maybe," she explains. "We use steroids to fight the inflammation, so sometimes people gain weight during treatment."

"OK, WAIT," I say. "Let me get this straight. I may lose — forever — my hair, my eyelashes and my eyebrows, but I will still have to pluck my mustache and beard, I'll have no short-term memory, my hearing and vision will diminish, I might have a weak heart and compromised lungs … and I could get fat?!"

"You'll be alive," she says. She continues talking about my slash-and-burn journey like it'll be a lovely stroll through a flower-filled minefield. Even before radiation has damaged my hearing, I don't hear anything else she says. I look at Jack and Don. They're looking at the doctor, moving their mouths and nodding their heads.

I slip into a fog, barely hearing the doctor's medical predictions if I do survive treatment. "Blah blah blah permanent short-term memory loss." "Blah blah blah lifelong hypothyroidism." "Blah blah blah weak heart." "Blah blah blah compromised lungs." "Blah blah blah poor vision." "Blah blah blah hearing loss." "Blah blah blah no hair."

And all I can think is maybe I'd rather die than live as a limping, bald, blind, deaf and dumb doughboy.

Leaving the oncology offices, I feel like this round of the game is complete, and I lost. Sensing my fear, Jack takes my hand. I think he's in as much of a state of shock as I am.

"You OK?" he asks.

"No," is my sole response.

My neck turns to wood and I develop a screaming headache. When we get home, I crash on the couch and sleep for several feverish hours.

"And this is exactly why you have to prepare yourself for what you're about to undergo," says Sue when I tell her how the appointment went. "I've called our friend in Canada. He and Al went to medical school together. He's one of North America's top integrative doctors advising Eastern treatments to complement Western protocols."

"What's the advantage of involving these Eastern treatments?" Jack asks.

I check out of the discussion and turn to my dog Arthur, petting him in long strokes. I'm finding the more we discuss treatments and my little, er, predicament, the less I want to hear. To my great surprise, I want to take a back seat in my treatment and let Jack drive. I want him to figure out what doctors I should see and what treatments I should undergo. I'm frankly too tired — and too distracted by my possible impending death — to remember names and places and dates and whether I should eat this or that or try this or that.

"Normally, he's very difficult to see, but we called him and told him about your case and he's willing to see you this weekend to help you design an integrative approach to your treatment," Sue continues. "But you'll have to travel to Salt Spring Island in Canada."

"Done," says Jack.

We visit one more brain tumor team in Seattle before heading to Canada.

Reputed to be the other brain tumor team that has risen to the top of Seattle's brain treatment cream, the Swedish Hospital doctors enters the room with a genuinely sympathetic demeanor. To me, they seem as soft and sweet as a bowl of chocolate pudding, peddling harsh information that I can swallow. They basically tell me all the stuff that the UW team told me, but their delivery is calming and peppered with warm smiles. Their outlook is upbeat and they too have handled medulloblastomas successfully.

They tell me my hair will grow back.

Even though they use photon therapy — not the highly-touted proton therapy — I decide to go with the Swedish team mainly because I like them and they seem so sweet, fueled by the fact that they too have successfully handled medullos. I feel like this is going to be a team that looks after my psyche as much as my brain and they would be the right battalion in a battle where good juju can be a comforting blanket in an ice storm.

CHAPTER 7

Sober news

Jack and I remain silent for much of our drive and ferry ride to Salt Spring Island to consult with the integrative doctor. Every so often I marvel, "I mean, is this too weird or what? Brain cancer? Me?"

It's been two weeks since the brain surgeon rang the death knell.

"I know," Jack nearly whispers. "It's so surreal ..."

We don't talk much. I feel like I should reminisce some of my favorite memories with him while we are privately settled in the car. But I can't think of any memories. My thinker has clocked out. And I think Jack just doesn't know what to talk about. "So you're dying. Yup. You're dying. Death. The Big D. Going going gone. Hello Pearly Gates. Say hi to your Dad for me"?

No. That wouldn't be a fun conversation.

So Jack drives in silence while I stare out the window pointing to the occasional hawk and flipping through radio stations, eventually resting my head against a pillow I brought and falling sound asleep.

As the crow flies, Salt Spring Island is 160 miles northwest of Seattle, in the Strait of Georgia near Vancouver, B.C. It's a bucolic wooded island with pocket farms, a quaint downtown, rugged beaches, quiet harbors and English-style gardens dotting the idyllic countryside. It's the kind of place that makes me wonder why I ever chose to live in a city. After being there only one day, I feel as if I've been there all my life and all that city stuff is just a grating memory.

Here, there is surely no cancer. I left all that ugliness back in Seattle for those city folk to wrangle. I devote my attention on the fresh air and the meandering roads bereft of traffic and the lack of hospital hallways and pinpricks and dirty news that brings me crashing to my knees. I decide to treat this weekend as a holiday. It's our well-earned break from my current beastly situation.

Jack and I peruse the Saturday farmers' market and settle into an intimate Italian restaurant overlooking the bay. This is so nice, I think, thoroughly exhausted from the drive. We order wine, and Jack takes my hands across the table. Why don't we do this all the time? I wonder. When was the last time Jack took my hands in his? Or when was the last time we traveled alone? Or when was the last time we even shared a romantic evening?

Our early years together were a lazy, sexy, blissful haze. I was a junior in college and Jack was traveling the country consulting for high-tech companies. After a brief hiatus from my initial alma mater, Smith College, Jack encouraged me to return to the East Coast for my final two years of college. I did return to Smith, but I was hardly interested in classes on Chaucer and discrete mathematics. The stale classrooms, monotonous lectures and brutal tests couldn't rival the fierce fresh love that loomed at the end of each week. On Fridays, I would board a bus to Vermont where Jack was working. Weekends were reserved for indulging in a tangle of affection and entwining in one another's newfound love. During my long winter break, he would head to work each morning while I snuggled in the wood cabin he was renting and read Tolstoy as the snow blanketed the fields around our intimate world.

During this time, I started to explore the notion of 'cooking.' When Jack returned after 12 hours of testing aerospace software, I would greet him with a martini and a colossally horrible concoction of burnt fried chicken or nearly raw steaks in a sticky wine sauce, which he would choke down with many sips of gin followed by many dishonest compliments.

I studied belly dancing at school for six months to surprise him with a personal erotic dance. Donning the large satiny polyester bloomers that I'd sewn and a swimming suit top, I yelled from the bathroom, "OK, push the button!" Jack pressed 'play' on our CD player. As an Eastern musical groove perfumed the air, I sashayed out of the tiny bathroom, ringing miniature tambourines strapped to my fingers, spinning around in circles, and bumping my hips in awkward convulsions.

Jack burst out laughing … and my heart fell.

"Oh, that's good," he guffawed. "You're killin' me."

No! I thought to myself. *This is the dance of the seven veils and I am your exotic seductress. This isn't supposed to be funny*!

So I finished the dance while he grinned. When the last sitar chord played and the room went silent, Jack clapped. "That was great. You are so cute, honey. I think the spaghetti's ready."

I went back into the bathroom and put my sweats back on — more than a little hurt that I actually thought he would be so be-guiled by my fervid performance that he would swoop me up and carry me to the bedroom.

Looking back, I don't know why I felt the need to be anything —
or anyone — but myself. As I watched his boss pull a long blond hair
out of one of the crabcakes I'd labored over for my first dinner party,
I realized I would never be a chef in the kitchen or a courtesan spy
or a Cape Cod socialite. I would always be my bungling gangly self
tripping on curbs and denting his cars — and that was what he loved.
He'd proposed to me six months after we met, putting me in the
throes of planning my wedding during my junior year at Smith.

After getting married, I graduated, and Jack and I set our sights
on traveling the world. We played around with the Peace Corps
(ultimately turning down their offer — long irritating story). While
Jack took a contract in Phoenix, I taught English in Japan for a few
months to suss out the possibility of living there together. Feeling like
Queen Kong stomping though the oceans of pointing and staring
crowds (remember, I'm 5 foot 11 inches), we decided we were just too
big (Jack's 6 foot 5) to live in a nation of 20-square-foot apartments,
paper walls, and subways that we had to crouch in to fit.

We settled on Brussels, where Jack had been accepted to Boston
University's MIS program in Belgium. That time was a mixed bag.
I could not for the life of me get a job — and having just graduated
college, I was busting to break the glass ceiling and hurtle to great
heights. Doing what, I did not know, as is the plague of many graduates with an English degree and a math minor. As our meager savings
dwindled, I took comfort in my new best friend, Abby, the only other
wife of the students in the graduate program. Still, the rich adventure
of living in Europe was a dream and Jack and our desperate love for
each other was still on the forefront.

When we returned to the U.S., we both secured jobs. Jack worked
for Paccar and I took a job at a small newspaper writing wedding
announcements and obituaries (oh, and the calendar section, mustn't
forget the calendar section). And then I would say, the romance be-

gan to fade as 'real life' took over, with jobs, pregnancy, home-buying, parenthood, and bills upon bills upon bills.

Time worked its ugly little magic. As we pushed our way through middle-class lives — Jack working in high tech, I writing for various publications, and both of us juggling meals and pick up times for Rose at nanny's homes and eventually schools — a certain flaccid chill snuffed out our candle-it dinners and our weekends buried under the covers.

Twenty-five years later, I wonder, does it really take cancer to rekindle romance?

Apparently, it does.

Pondering the faded romance of our youthful beginnings, I sit next to Jack as we meander through wooded glens and along the water heading to our destination: The integrative Dr. P's clinic in the forest.

"You know what?" I ask Jack, who hasn't mentioned opening a restaurant since my diagnosis. "I really think you should open that restaurant."

"I thought you hated the idea," he reasons.

"No, I very specifically hated the dive bar you were looking at," I set him straight. "But if you really can get the money together and find a suitable location, I think it could be great."

"What if it fails?" he asks.

"You won't know until you try," I say, secretly thinking it would keep him preoccupied if I pass on. "If all else fails, it would be a hell of a lot of fun. Imagine … you a restaurateur!"

"We can't afford it."

"You could raise money by getting investors," I suggest.

"You really think so?" he asks. "Who would invest in a restaurant?"

"Lots of people," I continue. "High tech millionaires and real estate tycoons. You can't throw a dead cat in Seattle without hitting one of those. You don't want to work in high-tech the rest of your life. You hate it."

"God, I would love not to be locked to a keyboard and mouse," he says.

"Then do it," I say. "When we get back to Seattle we can go back to your beloved dive bar and see if the last offer went through. If it didn't, you can make an offer, or at least meet with the current owners to discuss the possibility. Maybe they'll fall in love with you and wait till you can raise the money?"

"That's not the way real estate works, Deirdre," he says, slightly irritated with my naïve notion that owners would just wait until he raised money. "It's not that simple."

"Why? What's not simple? Write a business plan. Call your rich friends. Call the owners. Buy the place. Fix it up. Hire a staff. Create a menu, and start smoking for realsies. You know what they say, 'Build it and they will come.' See? Simple. Just — bing badda bang."

"Well you've certainly changed your tune," he notes.

"No, I'm just realizing how short life is and if you want to do something you should just do it."

I can tell he's thinking hard on the idea as we park the car.

"Hello," says a thin man approaching our car. "You must be Jack and Deirdre."

Removing our shoes before entering the clinic's inner sanctum, we exchange pleasantries with this sprightly bearded gentleman. After settling into his office, Dr. P gets down to business.

"Do you know your protocol yet?" he asks.

I (now) know what protocol means, so I answer.

"No," I tell him. "We actually just picked our medical team before coming up here."

"It will include radiation and chemo, I presume," he surmises.

"Yes. Radiation and chemo," Jack informs him. I look out of the window at the heavily wooded surroundings, already disinterested in the foggy discussion of my situation.

"Deirdre, you're about to undergo a highly toxic treatment that in and of itself is dangerous," he warns me.

"Yes," I say, snapping back into the room.

"And the ultimate goal is to provide your body with the maximum support to receive this treatment."

"OK," I say. "What does that look like?"

He proceeds to recommend a regimen of vitamins and herbs: Vitamin D3, Kyolic garlic, probiotic capsules, ground flax, food-based B complex, turmeric, DoMatcha green tea powder, Golden Flower herbs, resveratrol.

"Jack, are you writing all this down?" I ask.

"Got it," says Jack, tapping on his phone.

Now, with your diet," he continues, "Try only to source organic foods."

I always assumed one goes organic because chemicals are bad and bad is bad and someone somewhere has produced more-than-flimsy evidence that there is some level of toxicity in the evil puppy-killing chemicals sprayed and injected into much of our food. And yes, that's true. But there's more …

Dr. P explains that inorganic fruits and veggies simply quit producing cancer-fighting agents because they don't need to — the chemicals do it for them. So, a regular blueberry — normally considered a great antioxidant for brain health — is less effective because it no longer produces its own high levels of antioxidants. In fact, he recommends organic heirloom foods, which have the promise of less hybridization than even plain old modern organic food that's allegedly chemical free (or chemical reduced).

And what should I eat in this New World Heirloom Organic Diet? Eight to ten servings of vegetables and fruits per day; avoid omega 6 oils (corn, soy, safflower, sunflower, cottonseed); stick to coconut oil, cold-pressed extra-virgin olive oil and organic butter; consume only organic, grass-fed meat and (free-range) eggs; buy organic dairy, such as yogurts and certain aged hard cheeses; include pomegranates and pomegranate juice in my regular diet; load up on garlic and broccoli (but don't cook for more than four minutes); include shiitake mushrooms in my dishes; drink two ounces of wheatgrass juice (fresh or frozen) on weekdays (or five out of seven days); have a daily miso-based vegetable soup with seaweed, shiitakes and tofu (this is for brain cancer, I know soy is not recommended for certain cancers so please don't use this list for your cancer — consult a physician); and only consume a maximum of three glasses of pinot noir a week.

Whoa, wait, hit the brakes, back up.

"I'm sorry, did you just say three glasses of pinot noir a week?" I ask, incredulously.

"Yes, three a week. Maximum," he confirms.

"Three a week?" I repeat.

"Three a week," he repeats.

"Three?" I verify.

"Three," he verifies.

"Okaaay, we may have a problem there," I tell him.

"Why?" he asks.

"Because, I drink," I admit.

"That's OK," he says. "Just don't have more than three glasses of pinot noir, which contains resveratrol, a week."

I look at Jack. He looks at me as if to say, "Good luck with that!"

"Alright, anything else?" I ask, wondering if this guy is legit.

"Everyday good habits, exercise, walk, spend time outside, drink a lot of water, avoid sugars and processed food, get plenty of rest," he advises. "Yoga's good. Massage is helpful. Acupuncture's great."

"Oy," I let out. The Eastern regime is beginning to sound as tedious as the Western regime. Three glasses of wine a week. As if. To pretend I still plan on playing his game, I ask, "Can you recommend an acupuncturist in Seattle?"

"Yes, there's a great one in Seattle who went to school with my wife years ago," he says. "I'll get you his information."

"Thanks," Jack chimes in.

The kind doctor invites us to meet his wife at their farm in the evening. So we say our adieus and return to our rental.

"OK, the wine thing," I say as soon as we are safely in the confines of our car, "I mean, really? Three glasses a week? Why drink at all then?"

"It's alright, we'll just do it. I'll do it with you," comforts Jack.

When we arrive at our Airbnb, Jack draws a hot bath for me in an oversized outdoor bathtub that overlooks the bay.

"I have a surprise for you," he says, leading me to the private deck. "I got you bubblebath too."

Now, normally I'm not a bath person, let alone an outdoor bath person. But my ever-present chills (peppered with intermittent hot-flashes) render this big bowl of steaming water into a beckoning pool of pleasure.

"Oh, honey..."

"Come on, we can bathe together," he says, pulling out another surprise — a bottle of champagne. "Just one glass. Remember, our drinking days have to end for now."

"Well, one little glass of bubbly can't hurt," I smile, taking off my dress. "After all, the protocol hasn't technically begun."

We soak, he rubs my feet, I rub his feet, we even share a fleeting kiss.

"Ready for a nap?" Jack asks as I rise out of the hot water that's now inciting a hot flash.

"Am I?!"

As I sink into the cool sheets, Jack opens a window, slides in next to me and wraps his arms around me.

"It's going to be OK," he comforts. "You're gonna be OK."

After a solid hour of rest, the sun begins to set. Somewhat reluc-tantly, we drag out of bed and pull our clothes back on. It's time to head to the doctor's, who has invited us for a sunset visit on their back patio overlooking goats and an expansive organic garden.

Because I can't imagine showing up at anyone's home without at least a bottle of wine, we pick up a lovely Pinot Noir on the way. As we join the lithe Dr. P and his middle-aged wife sporting long salt-and-pepper hair (and I suspect wearing a hemp tunic, but I can't con-firm this) in their home on a hill, Jack presents the wine to our kind host. He takes it. He puts it in a cupboard. He pours four glasses of pomegranate juice. He hands it to us. I look down at my drink and at hummus dip on the table and think, *This is gonna be a short visit.*

It's been three weeks now since we received 'the news,' and I'm acutely aware of the fact that the brain surgeon's prognosis was "one month to a year." That means I could literally die in a week. As I walk Arthur through neighborhoods and along beaches that I've walked thousands of times, I curse the Canadian geese gliding along Lake Washington.

You geese might outlive me, I think. Arthur runs to the beach to chase tennis balls with another dog that's swimming in the lake. When I try to bend over to pick up his ball, I fall to my knees.

"Are you OK?" asks a man who is also chucking balls for his dog.

"No," I answer. "I have brain cancer and I have no balance."

"Oh. Wow," he says, perhaps a titch embarrassed with the frank-ness of my declaration. "Would you like me to throw the ball for your dog?"

At that moment, that is the only thing I want to hear.

"Oh my god, that would be so nice," I almost tear up. "Yes."

"No prob!" he says, grabbing a wet ball that Arthur's dropped and winging it out into the placid water with my Chuckit.

When I feel like Arthur's had enough exercise, I try to rise from the ground where I've been sitting, but I immediately fall again.

"Here, let me help you up," the dogman says, extending his hand.

"Thank you," I say, holding back tears. I feel so pathetic. I can't even stand up without help.

"Do you want me to drive you home?" he asks.

And I do. I do want him to drive me home. But pride stops me from accepting.

"No, really that's so sweet of you, but I need the exercise."

"Are you sure?" he asks, tilting his head in doubt.

"Sure," I say, trying to reach for Arthur, who keeps running away from me because he doesn't want to leave the lake. "But I will let you put Arthur's leash back on and walk him to the top of the bank."

"Oh yeah, sure!" the kind man retorts, grabbing Arthur by the collar and dragging him away from the water.

I wobble home and wonder how much longer I'll be able to walk Arthur. My dizziness grows exponentially each day, and I'm beginning to feel a sense of urgency about beginning treatment. My tumor is fast-growing, and we've frittered away three weeks so far interviewing doctors and researching alternative care. I want to get this show on the road, and I'm excited as we head to the kind doctors who are creating my protocol. Fielding questions from Jack and my brother Don, the medical team goes over my extensive procedures that will (hopefully) save me from the fate of the brain surgeon's original projection. They say I will start photon radiation in a week, coupled with chemo.

I'm not exactly "happy" treatment is about to begin — I'm more restless. The ticking time bomb in my head is speeding up, and if I am going to survive, I know time is of the essence.

CHAPTER 8

Cluck cluck

The morning after our appointment with my chosen brain team, Jack's phone rings.

"Hello?" he answers. "Yeah … Yeah … OK, let me ask you this, if this were your wife, what would you do? OK. Really. Wow. That's pretty compelling. Hmm. OK. We may just go that way. I'll let you know. Listen, man, I really appreciate your honesty. You too. Alright. Bye."

What? What? I'm thinking.

"Who was that?" I ask.

Jack tells me it was Dr. X from the team we've chosen to work with. The warm-and-fuzzy-chocolate-pudding photon cancer team who tells me I'm going to go through a nuclear war and they're so sweet that I almost (almost) look forward to it.

"Well? What did he say?" I press on.

"He says a new study came out this morning that indicates proton therapy may actually do less exit damage and — because you're getting nuked from stem to stern — maybe we should go with the other team who uses a new proton therapy gantry in North Seattle."

"The slash-and-burn-you'll-never-get-your-hair-back team?" I ask.

"Yeah, that one," he says softly.

"But they make me feel so lost and hopeless. I need a team that will gather around me and make me feel happy and root for me," I say. "Everyone says a positive approach in fighting cancer boosts your chances of survival. The slash-and-burn team makes me feel like if I do survive, I'm going to end up like some bald fat man or a clucking scratching featherless chicken."

"They're job isn't to host a love-in," he reminds me. "Their job is to make you better. And if the opposing doctor says he would want to treat his wife with the newer machines, then that's enough for me. I say we go with proton therapy and the team at UW."

"Oh God, I don't know. Why did he call you? I was so ready to begin tomorrow with that team," I whine. "Shit."

"If this man, who's a specialist in brain tumors, would go with the other medical team's proton therapy instead of his own photon therapy, I would go with the proton treatment. I mean, he told me that a study came out today that indicates the proton therapy appears to do less long-term damage to other organs."

I look blankly at Jack. I feel completely incapable of making any decisions, especially this one.

"What would you do if this were Rose?" I ask.

"I would insist on proton therapy," Jack says, tearing up.

"OK," I finally agree. "But only if you let the other team know they scared the bejesus out of me and that's just not cool. I need them to be nicer."

"I'll make sure they get that feedback," Jack promises. "I'm gonna call them now and commit. You're sure you're OK?"

"Yeah, let's do it," I concede. "I can feel this thing growing by the day. I don't think we can sit around and pick our noses much longer."

Jack lifts his phone and starts dialing.

"Are you sure you don't want me to stay?" asks Rose. "I don't mind cancelling."

A blooming Anglophile, Rose's three favorite things in life are literature, museums and tea. She has been planning and saving for a trip to England all year. During this trip, she's going to stay with our summer housemate Saul's parents in the pastoral countryside of Somerset with her good friend Augusta. Then their travels will lead them to London, where the girls will stay with a college friend of mine.

"Honey, do you really want to watch me go through radiation and chemo?" I ask. "I would rather have you go and enjoy the time of your life and spare yourself witnessing the ick I'm about to go through."

"But, what if …" she trails off.

"I'm going to be fine," I assure her.

And I really believe this. I believe if there is a 1 percent chance of survival, I will be in that 1 percent. I have to believe this.

"I feel funny about it," she confesses.

"Don't. Go. Enjoy yourself. You're not leaving for a few weeks, so we can have some quality time before you leave, and when you get back, I will be through my initial treatment. Really."

I have officially let go of the declaration that I'm on a one-month schedule. Having learned I may have a 60 percent chance of surviving, I'm shifting gears from imminent doom to probable salvation.

"Wellll, OK," she gives in. "But if you change your mind — at all — and you want me to stay, I will."

"OK," I agree.

"I love you, Mama," Rose says, her large brown eyes tearing up.

"I know," I choke out. "I … love … you … sooooooo … much. I'm going to beat this … for you."

CHAPTER 9

Hello God, it's me Deirdre

I'm so tired of saying "brain cancer." It sounds so serious. OK, I know it is serious, but those very words elicit a strange response in my friends and family — as if each time I say "brain cancer" I slap them in the face. They get all sad and morose, which makes me feel sad and morose and God knows I don't need to feel any worse about my current situation. I simply don't want to spend this time around a bunch of Debbie Downers. I'm willing to accept my reality. I've lived a happy, fruitful life full of fun and laughter. As people react to our news, I feel the need to pick them up off the floor, brush them off, look them in the eye, and say, "It's OK." I don't want to subscribe to a 'woe is me' attitude. If this is my final lap, I want it to be like the rest of my life. I want to hold onto friends and family as I wobble around dizzying surroundings and wallow in love and laughter. But it's not my final run around the track — not with that inspiring 60 percent odd of survival. Shit, I feel like I have a higher chance of dying in a car crash than from a little plum-size tumor hogging my brain. I commit to that optimism. I have to. This is going to be the biggest fight I've ever fought, and from here on out, I've decided to be the female Rocky.

To that end, dear people, I decide to rebrand my battle with brain cancer so it's more user-friendly. I want to take the piss out of the doom-and-gloom phrase — brain cancer — and recast it so people can step into my world and not feel so intimidated.

From this point on, I am referring to my diagnosis as "Brain Candy." My reasoning being it's so much more fun to say you have Brain Candy at a party, making people think maybe they'd like some candy too, until they actually find out what it is.

Brain Candy exists in the ethereal but dangerous land of "Candyland." Candyland is full of woolly monsters and pink bunnies and sharp-tongued dragons and large clouds that you can catch and ride and relax while watching the world pass by.

This frightening and exhilarating land is split into regions: WooWooVille, (Eastern treatment) The Wild West, (Western treatment), The Black Forest (from which there is no return), and Return to Home (survival). In WooWooVille, you'll find hypnotists, shamans, apothecaries, massage parlors, acupuncturists, Reiki goddesses, chanting monks, fluffy kittens, chubby chefs, unabashed affection … and possibly salvation from the inevitable. In The Wild West, you'll find nuclear bombs, toxic poisons, MRI monsters, hard-edged practitioners, oncology nurses in white lab coats and hazmat suits, all trying to provide salvation from the inevitable. If you land in the Black Forest, you're dead. But if I'm lucky, I'll toss the dice and land on the "Return to Home" button and my final track will be along You-win-it-was-all-just-a-bad-memory Lane!

Candyland hosts a balance of yin and yang. Without the yin, the yang would be unbearably harsh and hurtful. But without the yang, the yin might lead you to the Black Forest.

So far, I've spent most of my time in the Wild West. But our recent trip to Canada (which is north of Candyland) led us to WooWooV-ille's Hope Valley.

Feel like you have a brain tumor after reading this? Good. That's what my brain feels like — existing in its own special place outside of 'reality.'

Welcome to my new world order.

I know I'm talking a big talk, like this is all fun and candy. But the truth is, I have very little energy these days — now three-and-a-half weeks into my diagnosis. My days — once occupied with meetings and social engagements and long walks — have been reduced to a sofa, watching "Today" and "Ellen" and "Bewitched" reruns under numerous blankets and increasingly shorter dog strolls.

When friends drop by, we bubble through our tears, and then I ask them about their spirituality. I'm obsessed with their spiritual beliefs. I want to make the Black Forest less scary. What if it's a universe so wondrous that actually landing there would be ironically lucky? What if it's some divine bliss? Being an agnostic, this is not what I was raised to believe. Spirituality and religion were scoffed at in my childhood home. My mother was raised a Mormon and my dad was raised a Methodist, but they both rejected their respective religions when they reached adulthood. They in turn taught my brothers and me that religion was a load of crock. Consequently, I never really considered any sort of existence beyond the here-and-now, even though I attended parochial schools. In high school, I just thought chapel was the time when you got to sing and not answer any questions and maybe secretly study for the upcoming chemistry test. But my here-and-now is potentially going to change very soon, and so for the first time in my life, I'm wondering, "What next?"

I had always been told that when we die, we return to blackness. End of scene. End of story. But somehow, now being so close to that heaving darkness, the end as just an end and nothing more isn't sitting right. If anything, it's a piss-poor cop-out in storytelling. My friend Lisa drops off a copy of "Proof of Heaven," (Simon and Schuster, 2012), a book about a neurosurgeon's near-death experience. I devour the tale of his journey, wanting to believe that life doesn't just fade to black when it's over. And it is with great relief that I read about his intriguing and beautiful journey flying over the earth with an angel on his shoulder while witnessing divine beauty and absorbing universal wisdom. I mean, that's something to look forward to!

Friends bring me religious DVDs and prayer blankets and literature from their respective belief systems. I'm fascinated that so many of my close friends are actually … wait for it … religious. We've never discussed their beliefs, probably because I just wasn't interested in 'The Beyond,' and all that God stuff seemed liked wishful thinking. But now, well, you know, now I kind of want to believe that it'll all be OK and I'm going somewhere fabulous and not just pfuffing into a black hole of nothingness. My friends' notions of heaven and reincarnation and moving on to be gods of their own planets intrigue and comfort me, if not convince me. In my own insouciant way, I decide to accept that yes, the end is nothing to be feared. I don't have to define it for myself or be completely convinced of the great beyond, I just have to embrace my own little brand of faith that the end 'here' is just the beginning of some unknown 'there.'

Pondering my vague but burgeoning Deirdre Faith, I slowly walk Arthur past familiar homes and parks. That said, I have pretty much demanded Jack picks up the rest of the domestic slack. And though I loathe whiners, it seems to be all I do anymore.

"Jack, can you get some fruit and tea at the store, pwity pwease?"

"Jackie," I say, pointing to my feet, "Rub pwease."

"Mr. Jack Man, can you take out the trash, and do the laundry, and unload the dishwasher, and fix the TV, and rake the yard, and …?" the list goes on. It's kind of fun being the baby.

Jack accommodates most of my requests from my new Command Central (the couch), though I suspect he thinks I'm just taking advantage of my diagnosis so I can sleep on the job. But after I ran into that pylon at two miles per hour in the Safeway parking lot, we've all accepted that for now, my driving days are over.

I'm eager to begin treatment with my new medical team, but I can't until the gantry — the radiation machine — has an opening. Apparently, it's a pretty popular place. Meanwhile, I'm getting dizzier by the day and I sense my tumor actually growing.

With my final final medical team in place and my protocol outlined, our insurance company is balking at going with this hyper-expensive, relatively new form of radiation. They're not convinced that I can't just go old-school with time-tested photon treatment (which allegedly includes a lot of damage to other organs from the exit rays). While Jack haggles with adjusters on the phone explaining that I must start treatment soon because my tumor is fast-growing and I'm deteriorating by the second, I turn my attention to WooWooVille.

Now, if there is one thing I hate, it's taking pills. Looking at the mountain of pills and tinctures we bought after visiting Dr. P. in Canada, I see nothing but choking and gagging hazards. And this will not just be once a day. I will take some things before I eat, some things after I eat, some things before going to bed — it's a daylong affair of tincture-drinking and pill-popping.

But wait, there's more. Dr. P also suggested a morning smoothie to really pack in the veggies. Perhaps second to my dislike of taking pills, is downing 'healthy' smoothies. I mean, I can handle an Orange Julius with sweet yogurt, frozen berries and maybe a banana tossed in for good health. But a smoothie with flax and omega oils and kale and spinach and beets and raw garlic and OH STOP ME! They turn my stomach just writing this.

But by God, I'm gonna do it even if I choke on that shit while swilling it down.

Next goal: A healthy diet, which means a trip to the organic grocery store. Jack and I stroll the store throwing fresh yams and garlic and tomatoes and chard and tiny organic steaks and miso soup into the cart. I linger with a pregnant mother bearing blond dreadlocks and tie-dye and off-gassing a certain *odeur naturelle* as we eye the only 'junk food' the store carries, bean chips, hummus, dark chocolate and sugarless granola. Even though I'm not hungry these days, I've never been much of a health food fan and all this clean fibrous vegan fare is invoking my trailer-trash yearnings for Top Ramen, cheese quesadillas, Reese's Peanut Butter Cups, and microwavable popcorn. I look at the pregnant woman and wonder if she's having the same cravings.

I gently lay three bottles of pinot noir in the cart.

"Hey, you can only have three glasses a week," Jack appears out of nowhere.

"Uh, that's when treatment starts," I snap. "Right now I can do whatever I want."

"And he said to cut back on red meats. What's this?" he asks, pulling the shriveled little grass-fed steaks out of the cart.

"He said it was OK if I didn't eat a bunch of meat — as long as it's organic and grass-fed!" I say, resenting this food cop posing as my husband. "Oh, what's that?" I ask rhetorically, pointing at the packaging. "Organic AND grass-fed!"

"God dammit, Deirdre," he erupts. "This isn't funny! This is your life!"

Pissed, he puts two of the wine bottles back on the shelf and returns the steaks to the cooler.

On the one hand, I think, *How sweet, he really cares.* On the other hand, I think, *Who is this domestic nazi?*

"Fine," I spit, as if it's not bad enough that I'M DYING! "I'll just go sit at the counter, and you do the shopping."

"Fine," he spits back.

"Fine!" I say, blowing out of my nose. "Sheesh," I utter under my breath and head to the deli counter full of quinoa salads and nut burgers. I have to resist shuddering when the tattooed man with a bull ring through his nose asks, "What can I get you?"

"Nothing," I bristle. "I just want to sit down. Is that OK???"

"Yeah, that's fine," he says, with — I sense — a little 'tude.

"Fine!" I firmly state, watching Jack inspect hormone-free organic yams.

On our way home, Jack receives a text.

"Jack, don't look at your phone while driving," I admonish, still a little peeved at the contents in our recycled bags in the trunk.

"It's from [our friend] Shafeen," he declares, like that makes it OK to text and drive. "He says his ex-wife wants to come work on you."

Our good friend, Shafeen's ex-wife, Raheena, has become an 'energy healer.' I've only met her once, but I figure, *What the hell?* Right now I don't have enough energy to fill a thimble and any help in that department is welcome. Once we're not driving, Jack texts Shafeen back and sets a date for her to come over.

Now, from what I understand, Reiki is all about energy flow. That's my Cliff Notes description, but I'm sure a quick click of The Google will yield much more helpful information than my bird-brained understanding of life stuff.

It's a warm night when this kindly doe-eyed acquaintance arrives. Raheena walks in and with a single sweep of the living room she announces, "Your feng shui is blocked."

I look down at my fly. It's zipped.

"The living room energy is blocked," she continues. "I know a consultant who can help you fix it."

Ohhh, right, I think. Then I think, *Oy. Another consultant. More money.*

"It would be nice if you could adjust the room before starting treatment," she continues, looking at my TV like it's a loaded gun. "It will help create a healing environment."

I invite her to join me on the (misplaced) sofa, and we begin chatting about this and that. After our pleasantries are satisfied, she goes quiet, dangling a pendulum-like object from her finger that circles through the air.

"I'm reading the energy in the house," she informs me.

"Oh," is all I can think to say. I want to blurt out, "Two babies died upstairs many years ago with previous families and Jimi Hendrix played guitar in our basement!!!" But somehow, I sense those fun factoids about our 1920s stucco home might not be relevant to her work.

She starts humming and clicking and then, she starts to cry.

I look at her wide-eyed, wondering if I should start crying too. I mean, I'm the one with cancer.

"Don't worry, I always cry during sessions. It's just part of my process as I read the energy in the room," she explains. "Is there somewhere in the house where you can lie down comfortably?" she asks.

"My bedroom? That's where I lie down comfortably every night," I say.

"That would be perfect," she says.

I lie on my bed and she starts floating her hands over my body, legs and feet while humming and clicking.

"Can you feel anything?" she asks me.

"No," I tell her honestly.

"May I place my hands on you?" she asks.

"Sure," I tell her.

She continues, now placing her hands on me and blowing and sneezing and in general making me want to open my eyes to see what she IS doing, when she asks me, "What color is your tumor?"

"White and black and gray," I say, because those are the colors in the MRI (turns out it's white and pink).

"What shape is it?" she continues.

"Cauliflower-shaped," I answer, because that's what shape it is in the MRI.

"How big is it?" she asks.

"More than one and a half centimeters," I say, because that's what size it is in the MRI. "Like, a plum," I add, from out of nowhere.

"What is its name?" she asks.

"Sara," I say.

WHAT? What did I just say? Where did that come from? Sara? No, I've been calling it *Mini Me* and *The Evil Parasitic Twin*. It doesn't get a name. Especially a name as sweet as Sara.

"What does Sara smell like?" she asks.

"Popcorn," I say.

DOUBLE WHAT??? Where are these statements coming from? I mean, they're just falling out of me. In fact, I don't even believe I'm saying them. Sara is.

"How does Sara feel?" she asks.

"She's embarrassed. She knows she's done the wrong thing and she can't undo it and now we're all in a terrible bind," I continue. "She's horrified."

OK. Now, what is all this channeling and speaking on my behalf? It's bad enough that 'Sara' is trying to take over my brain, but my speech too?

"I need you to befriend Sara and explain to her that she has to leave," explains my friend. "She is in the wrong place and she needs to find an appropriate place to go. She'll need your help, Deirdre."

And all of a sudden, I feel sorry for Sara. Here's this little set of me-cells who are all excited to join the party and spring to life, and I'm about to do everything in my power to nuke the hell out of her.

That's right. I feel sorry for Sara — my mother-clucking Grade 4 inoperable malignant brain tumor. Fack.

After she leaves, I tell Jack about the experience.

"Sara?" he asks. "I wonder why Sara?"

"I don't know, but this is queer. When my parents were naming me, they were choosing between Sara and Deirdre," I remember my mom telling me. "And since these are embryonic cells coming to life, it's like my brain is growing another brain. Sara is my parasitic twin — And I'm going to have to kill her."

"Didn't she just recommend that you ask … Sara … to leave?" he clarifies.

"Well, yeah, isn't that 'killing' her?" I ponder. "I mean, it's all semantics. Kill? Leave? What's the diff?"

"I don't know," he says frankly.

And in my mind, I reach out to Sara and very politely ask her to go.

After my visit with the talking tumor lady, I decided to give acupuncture a shot. I'd only ever had acupuncture once before for a herniated disc, and it was a train wreck. The acupuncturist would stick an arsenal of needles in me, wire them with an electrical current, and leave the room. After a few minutes, my 'chi' would open and the electrical current would course through my body as if I'd thrown a hairdryer in the bath. Unable to move and screaming for dear life, the acupuncturist would eventually amble in after several minutes of desperate cries and turn the switch off. Those treatments did nothing for my herniated disc — and worse — they left me with a bad taste in my mouth for acupuncture.

But I'm in Candyland, and in Candyland I'll try anything.

The acupuncturist that Dr. P from Canada recommended is a quiet gentleman named David, who sports a sweater vest and a tie. He shows me into a pale green room with large windows, hanging plants and simple furnishings. First, we talk. I'm a little manic telling him everything, from what I had for breakfast as a child to my foray into Candyland and the fears that engenders.

He listens silently, stroking his nose in thought.

"What I would like you to do, Deirdre," he gently says, "is have you remove everything but your undergarments and hop on the table under the blanket."

He leaves me to get situated and "hop" on the table. When he returns, he lightly takes my right wrist in his hands and ever-so-gently applies pressure to my inner wrist with his finger tips. He moves his fingertips up and around this sensitive area of my wrist.

"What are you doing?" I ask.

"Taking your pulses," he almost whispers.

"Pulses?" I ask. "Don't you mean pulse? I only have one heart," I remind him.

"You have 12 pulses, each one representing a different region of your energy," he explains.

OK, here we go, I think. *A fraud. Twelve pulses. Come on. My mom was a nurse. She never mentioned TWELVE pulses. Just one. The heartbeat pulse. One heart. One pulse.*

"Twelve, huh," I say, somewhat sarcastically. "That's funny. You funny guy."

After gently placing my hand down, he returns to his desk and writes down some notes. Then he consults a large tome.

"OK, Deirdre," he turns around, "Let's have you sit up and swing your legs off the edge of the table."

I do. He maps his fingers around my back, drawing red dots here and there.

"Now what are you doing?" I ask.

"Finding your points," he says, lighting incense, which he then uses to light small dobs of mugwort that he sticks to my skin with a drop of water. "Now, I'm going to warm your points with mugwort. This will make the areas more accepting of the needle. Tell me when the points get hot."

Oh, how very Harry Potter, I think. Mugwort. I wonder if he's going to pull out a wand to slay Dementors and keep me out of the Deathly Hallows? I'll have to ask him ...

"Hot," I say, feeling a burny bit on my back. "Hot."

After each point is sufficiently primed with mugwort, he deftly sinks a needle into them and immediately pulls them back out. The pain is nominal and when we're through, I sit up and ... drumroll please ... I feel great! I'm still dizzy, but I feel more energetic than I've felt in months, maybe even a year. And I feel a little high, like maybe I just took a tiny drag off someone's joint.

"How do you feel?" my cousin Ada, who's visiting from Albuquerque to help me, asks when I return to the waiting room.

"Oh my god," I tell her. "You've got to try that!"

I make my next appointment for one week later. I wish it were for tomorrow.

After my initial Reiki treatment that left me a little floaty and my first acupuncture treatment that I would describe as unexpectedly settling, I decide, I'm kinda loving my time in WooWooVille. Jack too has sipped the lemonade, making his own appointments for Reiki and acupuncture based on my glowing reviews.

He even decides to book me with another Reiki practitioner, one boasting a popular radio show who fetches more than $500 per hour-long session and with a months-long waiting list. As a lifelong engineer, Jack's never been one for alternative anything, let alone energy workers. We limit talking about the potential of my situation — it's just too hard. But I can tell he's shaken to his core — grasping at anything that might help, even things that three weeks ago he would have considered pure bunkum.

For a cool $575, he books the appointment with this energy guru. Because I'm no longer driving, my friend Paula takes me to my first consultation. The Reiki practitioner works out of her home, a clean and airy newer house on a street in a tony neighborhood in Kirkland. Paula notes that her street looks oddly similar to Wisteria Lane on "Desperate Housewives." It almost seems like we drive down the Reiki practitioner's street in slow-motion, with handsome men mowing lawns, golden retrievers jumping for sticks at half-speed, and mothers herding perfectly coiffed children, stopping to wave as we pass by.

"Wow," I comment. "I don't know if this is charming or creepy."

"It's creepy," Paula confirms.

The comfortable waiting room décor smacks of Macy's-furniture-floor-meets-feel-good condo art. Marie greets us and starts asking me a few vague questions. Similar to psychic readings I've had in the past, she starts talking about me as if she's known me my whole life, telling me that I'm in denial and that I'm very scared.

Fuck yeah I'm scared, I think. *I have a ticking bomb in my head.* But I haven't told her about my medical situation yet, so I'm vaguely impressed.

"Any questions?" she asks.

I ask Marie how she became a Reiki practitioner. A former oncology nurse, she tells me that her patients' bodies started speaking to her. *When my body speaks, it tends to clear the room,* I muse, *and with this new increase in raw food I'm consuming, my body is speaking a lot more lately!*

When she's sufficiently sussed out that I'm facing a difficult illness (with very little feedback from me), she directs me to her candle lit treatment room piped with unobtrusive easy listening music and a massage table. Wearing a designer outfit, pumps and sporting perfectly coiffed blond hair, I eye the forty-something traditionally attractive woman and I can't stop thinking of "Desperate Housewives."

I lie on her massage table, and she explains that we all have chakras, which are energy wheels, if you will, that reside in different body parts, like your pooper, your hoohaw, your tummy, your swallower, your breather and your thinker.

Marie starts placing hands on me and hovering over my lower sacred chakra and humming in some funny little bird-like way while making motions with her fingers over my body. Although I never told her I have Brain Candy, she announces she must go to my head, it's calling her.

She cradles my head in her hands and says, "You have a brain tumor."

BINGO!

"Yes," I answer.

Marie explains that she is going to "move things around in my brain," or whatever that particular chakra is called. I'm thinking, *Is she going to slide the cerebellum next to the window and put some new curtains on the frontal lobe?* And as I'm making jokes in my head and Marie's "moving things around," she announces that a woman has entered the room.

She's petite, well-dressed, blond, and one of my grandmothers, Marie tells me. And I think, *Oh, that is just cheap bringing my grandma Rosemary to this situation. Just stab me in the heart already.*

And I start to cry.

And cry.

And cry.

I'm not crying out of sadness. I'm crying because I'm so touched, even happy, that my darling grandmother Rose could be in the room with me.

"She wants you to know that she has flowers waiting for you, but she doesn't want you to claim them yet," says Marie. "Oh, now she's kissing you on the cheek."

Then, Marie says, "A gentleman has just joined us. He's very large and has a white beard and he's related to the lady. He's holding her hand."

And now, I really lose it.

"That's my dad," I say.

"He's kissing you on the back of your head," she continues.

My father — with whom I was very close — had died nine months ago.

"He left so he wouldn't have to watch you go through all this. He was very worried about you and scared for you," she says. "He loves you very much."

My eyes swell shut and a stream of snot pours onto the carpet beneath my face, which is slung in the head cradle of the massage table.

"I love him too," I choke out, so overcome am I that my father AND my grandmother might be in the room with me now.

And so it goes. Marie does some interior design on my chakras, humming and chirping to her unseen world, moving energy around and adjusting the feng shui in my head. Fred and Rose attend the housewarming. I cry through most of the hour. And when she announces we're finished, I feel strangely serene in my new digs.

As Paula and I drive home, my friend Andrea calls me on my cell phone to discuss 'the situation.'

"If there's anything we can do …" she offers.

"Actually, there is," I tell her.

All of a sudden I have a hankering to go to church or temple or synagogue or just anywhere that hosts a faith-based community and believes in a life after death — be it heaven or reincarnation or whatever — I just don't want to fade to black.

"Can I go to temple with you guys?" I ask Andrea. She and her husband Darryl are Buddhists. They're hip, cool, smart people. I sense they will introduce me to a scene that I will find engaging without being over-proselytizing.

"You want to go to temple with us?" she asks incredulously.

"Yeah. I do."

"Darryl," she shouts, "Deirdre wants to go to temple with us."

"Deirdre?" I hear him say.

"Yeah, Deirdre," she confirms.

"This is so cool, we'd love to take you to temple," she comes back on the line. "Actually, there's a chant this Friday, do you wanna come to that?"

"Yes," I say, "I'll bring Rose and Jack too."

Saul, who is still living in our basement and exploring the Seattle area, joins the group. Having studied Chinese in school, he is inherently interested in Eastern religions. And Rosemary is delicately exploring Buddhism herself, beginning with a tiny altar in her room. We all trundle off to a community center where services are held each Friday. In a large auditorium, people sit on the stage/altar with a striking golden panel in the back. Everyone is dressed casually and smattered about the large room sitting on metal chairs.

There is a low hum of chanting echoing throughout the large room. Andrea hands us each a chant book, but it's not in English and they're going so fast I can't begin to find where they're chanting and try to chant along.

I find the words "Nam myoho renge kyo," which seems to be a regular chorus that the chanting refers back to and repeats often. I try to join in. It's impossible. Everyone is chanting this tongue twister in triple time. I look at Darryl. He's just a-chantin' away. I look at Rose. She and Saul and Jack are looking forward, spacing out to the hypnotic chant.

I resign myself to listen to the rhythmic utterances and try to take my soul to a place of calm, comfort and beauty, making a pact with myself to practice the chanting when I get home and to explore this notion of life after life.

My mind wanders as the rhythmic chants echo in my brain. OK, if I do die — which of course some day I will, if not this month — will I meet those who have passed before me and get to design my next life in front of some *nam myoho renge kyo* angel monk? I like this idea. It's a very comforting idea. And while I'm crafting the next iteration of Deirdre, I think, *what would I change? Maybe I'd give myself musical talent or design myself as a ballerina or choose to be a doctor — or better yet — become an international spy with all the glamorous intensity of a James Bond movie.*

Will I get to hang out with loved ones of yore, including my beloved cat Tu who just disappeared one day when I was 12, or Bugsy who was hit by a car in front of my very eyes soon after the disappearance of Tu? Will my dear friends Kirsten and Maia, who died untimely deaths at 35 from a blood clot and cancer find me so we can indulge in catch-up gossip? Will I get to hug my dad and smell the overbearing Old Spice that he wore?

After a good 20 minutes of group chanting and my head in the dazzling clouds, the service leads to a sermon of sorts. People step on stage one by one and start speaking like Charlie Brown's teacher "Wah wah, wah wah wah wah wah wah," and I tune out. The chanting was so heavenly but the talking feels so human and flawed. They screen a documentary about the branch's history that smacks of propaganda and members get on stage to testify how the religion saved their lives. It's all a bit much for me. I tune out the rest of the service, whispering *Nam myoho renge kyo* to myself.

CHAPTER 10

Adios. Au Revoir. Auf Wiedersehen.

Now that I'm no longer driving and I haven't the energy to cook a meal or even go out to eat, my dear friend Abby picks up on this challenge in my new life. Food. Abby is a widower and she's familiar with the hollow eyes of Jack and Rose, who are caught completely off guard by my newfound inability to do anything more than take a shower or climb the stairs to bed.

"How do you feel about doing a meal train?" Abby asks.

"What's a 'meal train'?" I ask her.

"It's where people sign up to bring you food so you don't have to worry about shopping and cooking during treatment," she explains. "My friends did one for us when Arron died. They're super helpful."

"You mean, people bring us dinner every day?" I ask. This sounds too good to be true.

"Yeah," she continues. "And we can tell them to prepare foods according to your doctor's orders — so they'll bring organic, home-made dishes. It's really a lifesaver."

"Where do I sign up?" I ask, glowing with the notion that I will be released from kitchen duty during this time.

"You don't Cinderella, others do," she laughs. "I'll get it rolling for you so you won't have to lift a finger in the kitchen."

Abby sets up the meal train and I watch in wonder as close friends and mere acquaintances fill out an online calendar with meals they will bring us in a matter of a few short days.

"Check this out," says Jack, closing the front door. He's carrying a large heavy box that was delivered to our door. "It's addressed to you."

"Ooh, open it, open it," I say.

It is a mixer. More specifically, it is a mixer/juicer/slice/dicer/pulverizer/watch-your-fingers beast of an appliance. It can take any well-meaning whole food and render it senseless with the push of a button.

It is … a Vitamix (VITAMIX, VITAMIX, VITAMIX, imagine yelling it into a canyon).

"Whoa, crazy!" I exclaim. "Who sent it?"

"Kat and Mike," he says.

Kat and I met 17 years ago. She was helping launch Sidewalk, a lifestyle guide to restaurants, shops, parks, all sorts of stuff, which Microsoft sponsored. I applied for a job as Kat's assistant editor running the restaurant section. My interview with her was on a Friday and I was scheduled for Rose's birth a la C-section the following Monday. Kat and I had great chemistry and she decided to give me a shot, asking, "Can you start on Monday?"

"Well, I don't think so," I joked. "I'm having a baby on Monday."

Kat looked at my stomach and nodded her head.

"Right. How about Tuesday?" she asked — IN ALL SERIOUS-NESS!

I did end up taking the job, but Kat patiently waited a few weeks while I scrambled for child care and we worked out a schedule where I could work odd hours and out of my home when possible. The job didn't end up sticking (nor did Sidewalk), but our friendship did.

Now, this many years later, she researched cancer treatment when she heard the news and discovered that juicing and smoothies were great if you have cancer. So she organized (with contributions from other friends Neal, Mary, Shafeen and Carrie) to have a semi-month-ly organic delivery of fruits and vegetables that I could prep in my new, handy-dandy Vitamix.

You know how I feel about smoothies, but I think, maybe this will make it tolerable.

Between the juicer, the fresh fruit deliveries, and the meal train, I feel that even if I don't survive, I'll eat like a queen to the bitter end.

"Have you thought about cutting your hair?" my friend Paula asks.

"Cut it? Why would I want to cut it? I'm about to lose it," I ex-claim. "I want to hold on to what I have as long as possible."

"I'm just sayin'," she continues, "do you really want to watch long handfuls of hair going down the drain?"

As with all things Paula, her painfully honest wisdom starts to make sense. I really don't cherish the notion of clumps of long strands on my pillow, on the sofa, on my coat, in my car, swirling in the tub. It seems so much more palatable to see little hairs going down the drain, like Jack's stubble in the sink.

If I only have a month or so with my hair, my hair that will never grow back, why not just once have a cute, edgy, on-trend 'do? Suddenly, cutting my hair in anticipation of losing it seems to make all the sense in the world.

"OK, let's get appointments … together."

Within hours, she has booked us appointments at Vidal Sassoon. I decide to color my hair like a peacock with blues and greens and purples on my soon-to-be new 'do. After my color is finished, the designer takes over and starts clipping my bob as I watch three-inch whisps of hair float to the floor.

"Done," says the beautiful hairdresser, handing me a mirror. "What do you think?"

When I hold up the mirror and look at my assymetrical pixie with flashes of peacock colors, I wonder why I had never tried an edgy cut before. Following my mother's insistence that I was a blonde, I had religiously bleached my hair most of my adult life.

"I love it!" I bubble. "It's so … hot! Now I'm bummed all over again thinking it will soon be gone."

When I get home, Jack and Rose are in consensus.

"Mom, it's so cute," Rose says.

"It is," agrees Jack, who has always preferred my hair long. "I like it honey. It's cute."

That night, I have a dream that is so visceral, it wakes me up and I actually remember it. I haven't remembered a dream in probably 20 years. I often awake knowing I've just had a nightmare, but all I have is a sense of a dream. But this one is very clear. It is my first cancer dream.

It goes like this: I arrive for my first radiation session and the tech walks into the room with a HUGE loaf of bread.

"You'll have to go into the bathroom and insert this bread into your vagina," she instructs.

"Are you kidding?!" I ask, staring at the monstrous loaf. "Why?"

"To protect your 'cavity' while getting pelted by the rays," the tech matter-of-factly explains.

"But that will NEVER fit up my vagina," I tell her. "It's larger than Baby Huey."

"Well, figure it out," she coldly states. "Other patients manage."

So I take the HUGE loaf of bread into the bathroom and think, *No, wait, I have to hipstamatic this and text my friends that this is what I'm doing. They'll crack up.*

I take pictures of the beast, and somehow I destroy the loaf of bread while photographing it.

When I take the chunks of torn bread back out to the technician and apologize for ruining the bread, she says, "OK, we have a replacement, but you're making this harder on yourself."

Then said technician comes out with this 3-foot-by-2-foot by 1-foot multicolored dolphin-shaped loaf of bread and says, "Now you have to put this up your vagina!"

And I'm thinking, *Right. Now I have to shove a dolphin up my vagina. Of course. That makes perfect sense.*

The next night, I have another curious dream that is actually Part Two of the previous night's dream. In this dream, I'm walking to my first radiation appointment and my dear friend Rachel bumps into me at the hospital.

"Deirdre, whoa. You're having your period all over your dress," she tells me, looking at my backside. "Here, I have an extra dress in my bag (which of course makes sense because she IS a burlesque performer). Go into that bathroom and clean up."

I head into the stall and think, *I'll just take a quick tinkle before cleaning up.*

I squat on the toilet, and what should come tumbling out of my vagina but … big multicolored croutons.

It's been more than two months since my initial diagnosis in May, largely because we dicked around so long picking a team, and once we did, the proton gantry didn't have any openings. The wait to begin treatment is putting me in somewhat of a panic. I can tell Sara's growing quickly as my symptoms intensify. Though I'm no longer counting down the days to my imminent demise, I know we have to get this show on the road. When people ask me why we haven't started treatment yet, I just sputter about photon versus proton therapy and this thing called a radiation gantry that's fully booked at the moment and I'm on a waiting list and — you know — *What do you think happens after death?*

I adhere to my daily walks with Arthur as per the WooWoo doctor's advice. We're maintaining a clean diet, though I haven't reduced my alcohol intake to three pinot noirs a week. I make regular appointments for acupuncture and I get a weekly massage. Rose manages to spend as much time with me as she can bear and I visit

Kathy as often as I can hustle a ride from someone who's willing to sit in a home for dementia while I coo over my mom. Jack, still on edge (much more than me) remembers to kiss me and say, "I love you" every day, and our house has become a train station of visitors who want to spend as much time with me before I'm quite possibly gone.

Friends and family from out of town book tickets to Seattle to come and help once treatment begins.

Ironically, I'm enjoying Candyland, except for the shadow of potential doom that looms in The Black Forest, which I patently try to ignore.

But all good things come to an end and we get the call: The gantry is available and my radiation is set to begin in less than a week on August 7, just days after Rose will leave for England.

Before I begin radiation, however, there is prep work to create a shell of sorts so that I can't wiggle one millimeter while getting blasted.

As we turn into the Proton Center for my "fitting," Jack and I note that there's a cemetery across the street from the center.

"I wonder if they offer package deals?" I joke. "You know … just in case."

Jack doesn't laugh.

Once inside the plush lobby, I make a beeline for a large chair in front of the fire. A team of techs will create a personalized shell to lock me into the table while I receive treatment. First, they warm a sheet of flat plastic mesh and then lay it over my face until it hardens in the exact shape of my face. That will lock my head into position, they explain.

After they complete the head cage (think Hannibal Lecter, only creepier) they stuff a gooey substance into my ears that hardens to the shape of my inner and outer ears to "fill the blank space" so the radiation doesn't hit an air pocket. As they're filling my voids, it occurs to me that it's kind of like the bread loaf in my dream.

Then I ask my real-life technicians, "Hey, do you have to fill vaginas when ladies are getting blasted down there to protect them?"

"Yes," they say. "The vas deferen, too, for prostate radiation."

HELLO! I burst out laughing, thinking, *It wasn't a dream. It was a premonition*!!!!

Next they put a blue beanbag type pillow under my body, which they then suck all of the air out of, and it shrinks around my body, creating a case of sorts in which my body will be locked during treatment.

"You know about the tattoos, don't you?" one of the techs asks.

"The tattoos?" I ask back.

"Yeah," she says, pulling out a needle and pulling my gown up to expose my belly. "We have to place six dots on your torso so we can align them with lasers and position your body in the exact same spot during each treatment."

"Can't you just … use a Sharpie?" I ask.

"It needs to be permanent so it's always in the same exact spots," she says. "OK, deep breath, here goes …"

She sinks the needle in my right rib and my vow to never get a tattoo flies out of the fifteen-foot concrete wall.

This is it, I'm thinking. *This shit is getting real.*

When we get home, I assess my pretreatment plan. Like parents taking prenatal classes so they can 'do childbirth correctly,' I want to 'do cancer correctly.' I still have the occasional doubt about the WooWoo lifestyle. I do, however, want to feel like I've dotted all my i's and crossed all my t's before jumping off the cliff.

My to-do list reads like this:

Closet/drawers: Clean.

Obit: I didn't finish writing it because I'm hoping to live and that just felt a little too creepy writing about my death.

Herbal therapy: Started. Hate it. Hate the pills.

Dietary changes: Downing one chard smoothie or garlic juice daily (not enjoying).

Food: Meal train starting starting with the first day of radiation.

Exercise: I guess I'll just keep walking Arthur. He was Mom's personal trainer, hiking buddy and quiet companion — he's good at it — I trust him with the job.

Acupuncture: Visiting David weekly. Loving it. Can't qualify what it's doing, but I swear I feel floaty, maybe less stressed, after each session.

Hypnotherapy: Relax, relax, relax. My friend Sue who is a counselor has made me a couple of personalized recordings to listen to that will help me maintain my strength and receive my oncoming treatment.

Spirit: When my brain starts looping on my Brain Candy, I've started chanting regularly to interrupt the obsessing. Plus, friends continue to drop by and share their spiritual beliefs, which I find very calming, if not completely convincing. A church group in New Mexico (that I don't even know) has made me a prayer blanket. Some nuns in Texas have written me a card with their prayers. One friend brings me her literature on Christian Science. Another friend brings me a video about her family's faith. A kindly Sikh gentleman has invited me to join their yoga practice. Before my diagnosis I would have been highly irritated by all this spiritual mumbo jumbo. Now, I find it comforting.

Reducing my alcoholic intake: Uh, hello! Treatment doesn't start for a few days! What're you, crazy?

Radiation fitting: (with tattoos, which is still pissing me off): Check.

Visiting Mom: I've warned friends and family that I will be begging, borrowing and stealing rides from them to see her. They're on board.

Rose: She's leaving for England today, so I won't have to worry about her this month. At 17, she's old enough to tackle world travel *sans* Mom and Dad. I catch my breath as we watch her step into the security line at the airport.

If I do go, I think, *she'll make it through. She'll hurt, but she'll make it through.*

And then I bury that thought, smile, and wave goodbye to Rose as she walks through security.

Jack: I'll need him, but he seems ready to serve.

Me: I hope and pray to an unknown power that all this preparation will help me move through this ordeal effortlessly.

With everything locked and loaded, there's only one thing left to do before treatment begins.

Throw a party.

If I'm going to have somebody entertaining my pre-treatment party — if only in spirit — I want it to be in celebration of, and thanks to, Mr. Welk.

I love Lawrence Welk.

He is my guilty pleasure.

I love the cheesy chiffon gowns. I love the redonkulously puffy hairdos. I love the sappy sentimentalism. I love the surreal serenity. I love the floaty dancing. I love Lawrence's crazy provincial accent. I just love it all.

When I was a child visiting my grandmother Rosemary for sleepovers in her dollhouse-like apartment in Wichita, she would prepare a small glazed ham and canned green beans for my brother and me. After what we perceived was the best cooking in the world, she would turn on the TV just in time for "The Lawrence Welk Show." Those nights were like holing up in a magical little kingdom for a whisper in time.

Lawrence Welk was our cruise director wielding his magic wand and he was my grandma's dream dance partner. In Welk World, there was no war or hunger or mean thoughts, or cancer.

Greeting guests in a blond bouffant wig and a tight pencil pink linen dress, I drink champagne with aplomb, dance through my dizziness to the polka band playing jigs in our back yard, pop bubbles flying out of the bubble machine we've rigged, unabashedly hug and kiss my loved ones, get ripped on booze, and celebrate in knowing that tonight is with us.

When the band plays an irreverent version of "So Long It's been Good to Know Ya," a few people recoil at the notion of dedicating that particular song to me on this night. I think it's hilarious and I sing along with them. I know I'll try to win this war, but there are no guarantees. I now take nothing for granted, neither life nor death, neither illness nor health. But just in case the next year doesn't resolve Sara, I raise my glass in celebration of today and echo the chorus.

So long, it's been good to know ya.

CHAPTER 11

Let the battle begin!

The proton therapy center is a lush modern-day structure north of Seattle. With its soaring window-encased foyer housing cozy overstuffed furnishings, compelling art, a latte bar, and a long gas fireplace filled with colored glass chips, the center feels more like a W Hotel than a medical facility. Feather-soft throws drape over chairs for the clientele, who, like me, tend to be cold. The staff greets you as you walk in with smiles and hugs.

Now, this is how Western med should be, I think, *like a trip to Club Med.* Only the clientele is not tan and bouncing around in the latest beachwear. They are thin and pale, some are gray, they're in wheelchairs and some sport brain helmets, underneath which there is no skull protecting their heads. The occasional swollen-faced bald child runs through the lobby to the playroom, seemingly unaware of his or her condition.

These are my people now.

I walk in with my niece Laura, who, as my inaugural radiation driver, has adorned her car's interior with Chinese lanterns and fresh flowers to cut the somber occasion with a light atmosphere.

After checking in and plunking down on one of the sofas, I put down my Brain Candy swag bag containing a thick robe and white slippers gifted to me (and all of their patients) by the center. I grab my purse and pull out my pills. Before each treatment, I've been instructed to take an anti-anxiety pill and an anti-nausea pill. I choke them down with a chai latte that Laura makes me at the latte bar … and we wait.

"Are you nervous?" Laura asks.

"No, just hungover from the party last night."

"Good. I mean, not good that you're hungover, but good that you're not nervous."

"Deirdre?" Brittany comes to me. I recognize her from my fitting. "Are you ready?"

"As ready as I'll ever be," I respond. "La, will you come back with me?"

"Of course," she says, taking my arm.

We walk into the inner sanctum of the proton therapy center. Past the nurse's station. Past the pediatric center. Past a couple of treatment rooms. The walls of each radiation therapy room are 10 to15 feet thick and made of concrete — just in case a random proton escapes. *Great*, I think, *and they're bombing those protons right into my brain and spine.*

"You can change in here and wait in this room when you're ready," Brittany instructs me.

"Here, can you hold my necklace?" I ask Laura, grateful not to be doing this alone.

"Of course," she says. "Don't forget your latte," she reminds me as we head for the waiting room.

"OK, Deirdre," says Brittany. "We're ready for you."

"Can Laura come with me?" I ask. Suddenly, I feel like a child getting my shots. I want my mommy there. But since my mommy can't be here, Laura is my next choice.

"Sure, Laura, you can see the gantry," says Brittany. "But during the actual treatment you'll have to wait in the lobby."

We enter the gantry. It's like a scene from "2001 A Space Odyssey." It's a large white room with a narrow table encased in a tunnel of sorts with a mammoth modern-day cannon that circles the bed. I climb up a small ladder into my body case that was made especially for me. They cover my body with blankets so I don't get cold and hold up the plastic mesh head brace.

"Are you ready for the mask?" Brittany asks.

"Ready? I've been waiting for this all my life," I joke.

"Before we lock you in, would you like to hear music during your session?" Nikki asks.

"Um, sure?" I answer, thinking my ears are completely plugged and wondering if I will even be able to hear music.

"What kind?" she asks.

"I don't know, pop?" I answer. I don't know why I say that. I don't even like pop music. But it's the only word I can think of related to music when she asks me.

"Done," says Brittany. "OK, we're going to secure the mask. Don't move. We'll position your head. Just hold perfectly still."

She and Nikki place the plastic mesh mask over my face and lock it down. It is so tight, I can't open my eyes or move my head even the slightest. The only things I can move are my tongue and my toes.

"This is so her head won't shift during treatment," I hear her say to Laura.

I can feel Laura's ick factor rising. I know it looks like some sort of medieval-torture-meets-"Star Wars" getup.

Next, they turn on lasers mapped to my tattoos, which is all programmed in a computer.

"These lasers have to line up with the tattooed dots on Deirdre's stomach to make sure she is in the EXACT position," Nikki continues explaining to Laura.

"Oh," is all she can choke out.

"OK, Laura. We're ready to start the X-rays to see if her position is set," Brittany tells her. "So you're welcome to wait in the lobby. We'll come get you when we're finished."

I hear Laura and the techs shuffling out. It's quiet for a few seconds that feel like hours.

"Alright, Deirdre," I hear on the loudspeaker. "We're ready to go. Hold absolutely still."

Now I hear the X-ray, which has opened above my head like a drawer out of the spaceship structure to take pictures. I try to open my eyes to see what's happening, but I can't. The head mask is too tight. In fact, the pressure is so great, my teeth are hurting.

The techs return over and over, moving my body an imperceptible titch here and there.

"We're gonna just shift you a little to the left," one will say as I feel them pushing on my body and pulling on the sheet beneath me. "Can you move your body up toward your head? OK, good, now can you stretch your neck really long pushing the top of your head toward the wall? OK, good."

It takes what seems like an eternity to align my body, and now my left shoulder is starting to ache where the body encasement presses on it. I wish I could open my eyes.

"Alright, Deirdre," I hear on the loudspeaker. A doorbell sound rings, which signals the staff to leave the room. The blast is coming. "You're good to go. Remember to hold absolutely still."

Then — I shit you not — Pandora pipes Imagine Dragons' song "Radioactive" into the speaker. And JUST as I hear a series of ominous-sounding low clicks and what sounds like horses banging at a gate, I sense the cannon pulling up to my head, I feel popping in my ears, I smell ozone, and I hear, "WHOA-OH-OH-OH-OH I'M RADIOACTIVE! RADIOACTIVE!"

Touche, I think. *Nice one, universe. Very funny.*

The radiation cannon (for lack of a better word) can swing around my table a full 360 degrees. It starts with the right side of my brain, then circles around to blast the left side of my brain. After finishing with my skull, the team re-X-rays my back to make sure I haven't moved before sliding the table closer to the wall in three successions, the cannon swinging underneath me to zap my cervical, thoracic and lumbar spine as the table shifts for each section of my back.

After more than two excruciating hours of lying bound on the table on my back, Nikki announces on the speaker, "OK, Deirdre. We're finished. Good job."

The team quickly removes the face mask, which is so tight it leaves a waffle-like grid on my cheeks, chin, nose and forehead. They extract me from the body case and help me sit up.

"How'd it go?" asks Laura, whom one of the techs has brought to the room.

"Great," I tell her. "I mean, it's creepy and lying still for a couple of hours is uncomfortable to say the least, but it isn't painful. In fact, I can't even feel the radiation … I just hear and smell it. One down — 30 to go!"

"Fabulous," she bubbles. "Why does it take so long?"

"They have to zap both sides of my brain and my entire spine, just in case any cells have crawled down my back," I explain. "And the positioning takes forever."

"Ewww, right," she says. "Any chance you feel like going for lunch?"

"You read my radioactive mind!"

When I get home, Jack hugs me and offers me a glass of pinot noir.

"Ya know, I'm not into it," I say, noticing the surprise in Jack's eyes. "I think I'm just going to abstain from alcohol during treatment. Maybe just go at this battle sober."

"You know, I'm glad to hear you say that," he says. "Good on ya."

The next morning I wake up and I can barely stand. I weave my way into the bathroom, practically crashing onto the toilet. As I weave back to my bedroom, I fall onto my bed. I am so weak I can barely sit up.

"Jack," I try to yell. "Jack!"

He comes to the bottom of the stairs and yells up, "Did you call me?"

"Help," is all I can muster.

"What's up?" he asks, coming into the bedroom.

"I need help getting dressed," I whisper.

"OK, OK," he says. "What do you want to wear?"

"My blue dress," I point to my closet. "And leggings," I point to the dresser.

We struggle through getting me dressed. I can barely lift my arms or legs.

"Can you help me get downstairs?" I ask. I feel so pathetic.

"Sure," he says. "Are you OK?"

"I'll be fine. I just need help."

Ada is taking me for radiation today. When we get to the facility, Ada escorts me in on her arm.

"Deirdre!" the receptionist greets me with a smile. "How are you feeling?"

"Weak," I say, scanning my patients-only badge and heading to the sofa. I swaddle myself in a blanket. Ada hands me a chai. I take my anti-nausea and anti-anxiety pills. Seth, another tech, comes out to collect me.

"Can you come with me, Ada?" I ask, still not wanting to get a shot without my mommy.

"Sure," she says, gently taking my arm.

Today, I'm happy to be strapped in. The thought of just lying there for two hours sounds like a welcome relief. No sitting. No standing. No talking. Just lying still.

I sleep through part of Round One. I don't even hear my pop music or the instructions from the techs. At one point, I start to cycle on my death again. I haven't done that in weeks, basically since the first oncologist I saw confirmed that I had a fighting chance. I think of Rose. She's leaving for England today to have the time of her life. I think of Kathy. She's struggling to understand where she is and why she's there. I think of Jack. He's working from home, probably working on his computer, and worrying about how weak I was this morning. I hear the doorbell rings and the loud thumping and the horses beating down the gate. I smell the protons frying my brain and making my ears pop. My shoulder hurts where the body case rubs, going from irritating to agonizing. My teeth hurt where the mask grips me hardest. After several hours, we finish. I need help crawling down the ladder from the table. I can barely walk. Ada takes my arm.

"I need to lie down," I whisper.

"What?" Ada asks, leaning into my face.

"Lie down ... I need to lie down," I can barely utter.

"Is she OK?" John, one of the techs, asks.

"Can she lie down?" Ada asks.

"Absolutely. Let's put her in a pediatric room."

I focus on the bed and fall into it.

"What's going on, Deirdre?" John, one of the techs, asks.

And I can't speak. *Oh god*, I think. *This is it. I'm dying. This is death. The mother-fucking radiation has killed me.*

"Let me get the doctor," John says.

In the distance I hear people shuffling around.

"I'm Dr. K, the pediatric oncologist," I hear.

"What's going on?' Ada asks.

"She just fell apart," someone chimes in. "She seemed fine when we started."

I feel someone take my vitals.

"Let's try an IV drip and see if she's dehydrated," someone else says.

I feel the needle sink into my arm. And it happens again. I feel my soul floating up, trying to pull away from all this. *No! No!* I think. After more time, I don't know how much, I hear the doctor suggest I go to the ER.

"Deirdre," somebody says into my ear, "We're going to send you to the ER. Can you walk to the car or should we call an ambulance?"

I know I have to answer. I gather all the strength I have and whisper: "Ambulance."

I hear Ada call Jack. Then I hear a rustle and sense the medics have arrived.

"Can you stand up ma'am?" somebody asks.

While I can hear them, I cannot respond. I feel my body being lifted onto a gurney.

The sirens scream as the ambulance pushes through traffic and neighborhoods. I try to open my eyes to look out the back-door window and see where we are. Every so often, I recognize the top of a building or an underpass or an intersection. My vision is completely blurry and it takes a monumental effort to open my eyes. The EMTs remove the gurney and push me into the ER, where, again they check my vitals and insert a new IV. The attending nurses and doctor ask me a series of questions, but I can no longer speak, so Jack, who has just arrived, answers on my behalf. I hear them tell Jack that my radiation oncologist is on her way and they'll be sending me for a CAT scan in the meantime. The gurney starts moving again.

"Deirdre," somebody says into my ear, "we're going to give you a CAT scan. It will only take a couple of minutes, then we're going to move you to a private room."

I say nothing.

"You're gonna be OK," the person tells me. I can feel my eyes crying. I am so happy this person tells me that. *I'm gonna be OK. I'm gonna be OK. Nam myoho renge kyo. I'm gonna be OK.*

While I sense the CAT scan clicking around my head, I try to will my soul to come back to me. *I'm gonna be OK,* I tell it. *Please come back to me. It's not my time. A voice told me I'm gonna be OK.*

After the scan is finished, I feel somebody wheel me through the hospital and into a room. I sense Jack and Ada are there.

"How'd it go?" Jack asks.

"I don't know," a voice says. "But I heard the doctor's on her way."

Somebody fusses with my IV.

"We're going to include some steroids in her drip," the voice tells Jack.

I hear others entering. Family. My niece Kimmie, and my brother Don. I feel them take my hand or kiss me and discuss the turn of events in hushed tones.

Then, apparently Jack enters the room.

"Hi, Jack," a woman's voice says. "So, what happened?"

"I don't know. Deirdre was super-weak this morning. I helped her get dressed, then Ada picked her up and took her to the proton center. Apparently, after Deirdre's treatment, Ada said Deirdre couldn't walk or talk."

"I've had a look at her," says the woman's voice. I realize this voice is my doctor. She sounds so nonchalant that I think everything must be OK and that I'm not dying. "She's had some swelling in her brain from the radiation. The steroids should bring that down. And we're hydrating her, as you can see. When was the last time she ate?"

"Yesterday," Jack tells her. "She didn't want breakfast this morning."

"Right," says the doctor. "I suspect she'll pull out of this before too long. The steroids are fast-acting. Then if you could get her to eat, that might not be a bad idea."

"So, are we canceling her radiation on Monday?" Ada, who followed the ambulance, asks.

"It's too soon to make that call," she says. "I'll come back later today to assess the situation. But if she makes a full recovery, I'd like to keep her on schedule."

"It just doesn't seem like she can handle it," Jack presses on.

"You know, this happens with patients," she tells him. "We usually don't see this until patients are three or four weeks into treatment, but it's rarely a show stopper. It's good that this happened on Friday. Deirdre will have the weekend to recover and hopefully by Monday she'll be ready to go again. OK?"

"I guess," says Jack, doubtfully.

"Alright," she says. "The team here will keep me updated throughout the day, and I'll swing by this evening to check on Deirdre. Because her reaction was so extreme I'd just like to keep her overnight so we can keep an eye on her."

"It's not like she's jumping up to go anywhere," says Jack. His voice is tense.

"She'll be fine," the doctor wraps up. "Let the steroids do their thing and she'll pull out of this. K?"

"Yeah. OK," he hesitates.

"Alright. I'll see you this evening," she says. "See if you can get her to eat."

"Yeah, bye."

"I have blueberries," somebody offers. "Do you want to see if she can eat?"

"Sure," Jack says. "D-D, want to try a blueberry?" I feel him rub one along my lips. I am hungry. I can't speak, but my mouth is slightly open and he drops one in. I try to chew, but I simply can't. I can't even close my mouth. Jack doesn't know I didn't chew it, so he pops another one in. Now I have two blueberries sitting on my tongue. He pops a third one in. Ach! I can't tell him to stop this. But when he goes for a fourth berry, an unknown force helps me say, "No," and close my mouth.

I fall into a deep sleep. When I wake up, I chew the now-mushy blueberries. I swallow them. Then I go back to sleep.

🍭 🍭 🍭

"Dad!" I say. "You've come to see me!"

Though he's been dead for 10 months, by some miracle my father has just walked into my hospital room. He's visiting me, and I'm sooooo happy to see him.

"Come here!" I tell him. "Come stand by my bed. Everybody, step aside so Dad can get through. Go on. Move!"

"What?" Jack asks. "D-D, what are you saying?"

"Who drove you here?" I ask as my father steps toward my side.

"Whoa. Deirdre, your dad's not here," Jack repeats.

"So you heard about my cancer?" I continue.

"OK, this is freaking me out," Kimmie, who has joined the group, says.

"Weird," Jack says.

"I think she's having a visitation," Kimmie reasons.

They're all being so odd, I think. *They should be saying, 'hi' to my dad!*

"Deirdre, you're hallucinating," Jack marvels.

Things blur out and my dad fades away. Now, I'm working on a long-neglected project.

"I want to paint the cupboards this way," I swipe my hands above me. "It will be beautiful with this soft white color. And let's move the stove over here to make room for a double refrigerator there."

"Deirdre, what are you talking about?" Jack asks.

You know how sometimes you have a bad dream and you realize that you're having the bad dream while you're still dreaming and you tell yourself to wake up to get out of the dream? Well, that's what this is like. I realize — while hallucinating — that I am hallucinating. And mid-hallucination, this unconscience/conscience realization makes me laugh.

And again, my soul snaps back into me like a rubber band. I know I am going to survive this rough patch. It's as if the laughter at my own hallucinations is bringing me back (though we know it is the steroids … or is it?). I open my eyes and see Jack, Ada, Don and Kimmie, and I laugh again.

"I was hallucinating!" I say.

"Oh my God." Jack tears up. "You're awake! You're talking! And yes, you were hallucinating! Oh, honey, hi!" He stands and kisses me. "How do you feel?"

"Fine," I nonchalantly say. "Tired, but fine."

"You scared the shit out of me!" he exclaims.

"I scared me too," I admit. "What was that all about? How embarrassing. I just went off the deep end."

"They think the radiation caused your brain to swell," he explains.

"I know, I could hear everything. I just couldn't respond," I tell him. "That was so weird. How long have we been here?"

"About five hours," Jack tells me. "Dr. H said the steroids would act quickly. Thank God you're OK."

"Hey, my dad visited me. It was so awesome," I tell them, radiantly happy. "And then I was making our kitchen so beautiful. We really have to redo our kitchen."

"Yes, we will eventually redo our kitchen," he laughs.

"With a double fridge?" I ask.

"With a double fridge."

The doctor releases me from the hospital the next morning, and I feel like nothing ever happened. After recuperating during the weekend from my, er, little breakdown, I decide I'm ready to go at it again on Monday.

I listen to the hypnotherapy tapes that Sue created for me, which are designed to help my body and soul receive the chemo and radiation with maximum ease and benefit.

I take my herbs.

I eat my healthy meal train food.

I walk friggin' Arthur two miles a day, up and down big hills.

I rest. Then I rest some more.

I watch comedies to keep my mood upbeat.

I hang out with friends and family (or rather, they hang out with me in my corporate headquarters known as "the family room sofa").

I get my acupuncture.

I throw in a massage.

I do not — repeat — do not drink.

And when my chemo oncologist says we're gonna wait on starting chemo till I'm completely stable, I say, "Ha! I ain't no house of cards! I'm the fucking Rock of Gibralter! Chemo? Bring it on Baby. Bring! It! On!"

To which he says, "No."

To which I say, "Suck it! I want the chemo. Gimme da chemo, beotch!"

To which he straightens his tie and says, "What did you just say?"

To which I blush and say, "Ohhh, rewind, erase ... brain cancer ... bad jokes ... actually, not even a joke, just too many episodes of "Orange is the New Black" .... no chemo for now ... got it."

Life has eased into a sort of slow-motion slightly surreal montage. It's like I'm following my own little path in Candyland bumping into other players on the way.

I have quit drinking altogether (miracle of all miracles). I have quit going out at night, which is huge because I routinely go to burlesque shows and other live shows in Seattle. Ada, who plans to move here from Albuquerque to help me all the way through this ordeal, organizes the flow of friends who want to make sure they squeeze in some D-D time ... just in case. Meal train becomes my connection to the outside world as the sweetest team of gourmet buddies delivers fresh veggie lasagna and sweet potato puree and heirloom tomatoes and goat cheese salads and homemade organic curry chicken and creamed spinach — much of which is prepared with the late summer harvest from their gardens. Neighbors drop by to walk Arthur with me. Leslie, my neighbor across the street, leaves funny cards of encouragement on our front porch every day.

Another friend, Annette, organizes Team Deirdre to help raise money for brain cancer research in a walk around Seattle Center. A professional artist, Annette creates hilarious "Team Deirdre" lanyards with my face superimposed onto a featherless chicken. I join the walk with my friends (who all dutifully wear their lanyards). Entering the square filled with other teams who carry placards dedicated to lost loved ones and loved ones currently struggling with brain cancer brings me to my knees. *There are so many of us,* I think, *some who lost, some who will make it, some who won't.*

And then I read a daunting statistic from the American Cancer Society: One in three American women will develop some form of cancer during their lives, and one in two American men will.

Walking around Seattle Center making small talk with my team as I clutch various people's arms, I can't help but shudder at the epidemic plaguing not only those around me, but so many future players in the game of Candyland.

CHAPTER 12

Hair today, gone tomorrow

Do you ever have one of those days where you think, "I'd rather be sick than go to work" or, "Kill me now, so I can miss that test tomorrow"?

Well, I have. Lots of times. And though I really loved my pre-cancer life of making little documentaries and writing the occasional article, I was tired. Tired of the daily grind to get it all done, from work to family to fun.

Yes I'm weak and dizzy, but in a twisted way, I'm enjoying my new life. I'm enjoying the fact that I don't have to get up early. I'm enjoying the fact that I have zero responsibilities but to try to live. I'm enjoying the fact that — for now — I'm off the hook, from helping Rose grow up, from returning a million emails and phone calls for my latest film, from taking our car in for oil changes on my way to Costco or the post office or the bank or from tending to whatever the fuck little mundane tasks weigh down my days, weeks and months. My conventional life has had to take a back seat to my complete and total self-care. It's selfish, I know. But there you have it. I'm not really suffering through this, I'm experiencing it. Even when I meet people on the street, they're surprised to learn of my current situation. "You look great," they say. "I never woulda known."

And yet I wonder, *now that my medical team and I decide that I'm stable enough to start chemo, will my newfound life take a turn for the worse? Will I lose 1,000 pounds and turn gray and flop around like a dying fish?*

I recall my chemo oncologist's words at one of our appointments. "It's best to visualize this as war. Take no prisoners. Kill all enemies. This is something we can try to fight."

Try, I think. *Try? Watch this bitch. I'm gonna kill it!*

At the end of August, during my third week of radiation, Dr. C feels I'm stable enough to start my weekly chemo pushes, which I was supposed to have started during my first week of radiation.

As I take the elevator to the chemo ward on the eighth floor, I expect to hear people crying and vomiting and basically suffering untold cruelties. But as I enter, the only thing that stands out is a sign that this is a "scent-free zone" and a series of curtained-off areas.

I try to sneak a peek at the other chemo patients to see where I'm headed. They're mostly bald and in varying stages of health, but nothing dramatic and scary.

My tech seats me in my own little section and starts me on an IV drip. They'll hydrate me first and then administer the "push," which is a 15-minute injection containing two mg of Vincristine (derived from the periwinkle flower) through a vein in my arm. The whole process will take less than two hours. But from what I've read, getting chemo is one part of any cancer protocol that brings patients to their knees.

You'll be OK, I tell myself, *after all, you listened to your hypnotherapy tape this morning that will help you receive your treatment with maximum benefit. You drank your foul smoothie. You had acupuncture. You walked and all that other stuff. You did your homework.*

As I'm waiting for my chemo drug to be approved by someone, somewhere, there's a middle-aged man sitting across from me. He has all his hair.

"Nurse," he calls. He is surrounded by family.

"Yes," the nurse stops.

"Can I have an ashtray?" the cancer patient asks.

"I'm sorry?" she asks, somewhat surprised.

"An ashtray," he reiterates.

"Um, there's no smoking allowed in the hospital," she says.

And I'm thinking, *Really? He's on a chemo ward in a hospital and he's asking for an ashtray? This is delicious.*

"If you want to have a cigarette, you'll have to leave the campus," she explains. "A lot of people smoke in front of the hospital at the bus stop. But you'll have to wait until your chemo is finished."

"Oh," is all he says, disappointed.

Delighting in this grand display of the most outrageous request, I wait for my chemo.

"Here we go," says my oncology nurse carrying a small plastic bag marked, "CHEMO."

The nurse puts on goggles and a disposable hazmat suit.

You read correctly: Goggles and a hazmat suit.

"Why do you have to wear that?" I ask.

"We can't get any of the chemo on us," he responds. "It's very toxic."

"Wait, you're wearing a hazmat suit, but you're pumping the very toxic poison directly into my veins?" I ask with a fake smile on my face.

"Yes," is all he says.

And then I think of the radiation center, with its fifteen-foot-thick concrete walls and the radiation that they send right to my brain and down my spine.

"That which doesn't kill you makes you stronger?" I say/ask/ think.

"Right," he says, also wearing a smile on his face. "Ready?" he asks, after checking and double-checking that I am indeed Deirdre Timmons, born 5/21/66.

"What do I do?" I ask.

"Nothing," he says. "I'll just inject the chemo slowly into your IV feed, like this," he says, slowly, gently, pushing the poison into the tube feeding into my vein. "This is why it's called a 'push' infusion," he explains. "Because I'm literally pushing the chemo into your IV. And ... done," he says, pulling the empty syringe out of the tube after about 15 minutes. "When the saline drip has finished, you can go home."

He tosses my spent syringe in a hazmat receptacle. He tosses his hazmat garments into a different hazmat receptacle, and he removes his goggles.

All clear!

There is: No throwing up. No coding. No golden light. No watching medicos revive me from the corner of the room. I didn't even feel the IV come out.

"Will I get sick from this?" I ask the very kind man.

"Honestly? Probably not," he smilingly tells me. "Your biggest side effect will most likely be constipation, maybe some dizziness, and you might get a little fuzzy headed."

Grrrrr, I think.

"I already have all those symptoms," I explain. "Can't I have something impressive and new and cancery?"

"Don't hope for that," he says.

So for now, I'll go in once a week for my chemo "push," which is supposed to interrupt cancer cells' ability to reproduce and act as a "radio sensitizer," which is a very fancy way of saying the chemo makes the radiation more effective.

Ah ah ah ah ah ah oh ai-y-ai. Push it real good.

It was inevitable.

Less than a week into chemo and 21 days into radiation, I wake up and notice my pillow is covered in blue, brown, green and purple strands of hair. I take a deep breath, for I know that soon my cute little peacock-colored pixie will be no more and I will be sporting a chemo chrome dome.

"Jack," I say, waking him up. "Look at my pillow."

"There it is," he states flatly. "Enjoy it while it lasts."

I run my hand through my cute new pixie, and with one swipe, my scalp yields an entire fistful of hair. I thought I'd be mournful when I hit this stage. But oddly, I'm fascinated. I roam around the house all day, pulling at my scalp and showing off my harvest to anyone who will look. At night, a collection of people drop by my house and I assault them with my show.

"Look what I can do," I insanely show them. Then I pull out a big handful of hair, not quite impressing anyone, but making plenty of them gag.

That is, until Paula comes over.

"Oh, let's have a hair-pulling party and see if we can pull it all out," she gleefully says, grabbing at my scalp and pulling out yet another handful. "Here, let me film it!" She pulls out her iPhone and coerces me (trust me, it wasn't hard) to yank out tufts of hair on camera. Robert, our friend, joins in.

"Do you think if I ride in Robert's convertible, the air will blow it all out in one ride?" I ask. "We could film it! That would go viral on YouTube — start the ride with a head of hair, end the ride bald!"

"First let's see what the blow-dryer does," Paula reasons, ever the pragmatic show producer.

We're all disappointed to see that it's not falling out that readily, so we abandon the convertible plan and just return to our seven-year-old mentalities of pulling it out by hand. We fashion different mustaches out of the fresh handfuls of hair and click photos of each other: "Sieg Heil!" I say, extending my hand in a Nazi salute. "Hey, Mr. Kotter!" I call out with a bushy '70s 'stache. "Obey Fu Manchu or every living being will die!" I scream with my Manchu upper lip.

We cackle and laugh.

Jack sits in the other room, watching quietly.

The sick humor helps me make light of this heinous development. It is my coping mechanism, if you will. I'm looking down and just putting one foot in front of the other, trying to ignore the wasteland that my life has become and keep a smile on my face. But Jack finds no humor in our situation. He's looking at the horizon — and it's scaring the shit out of him.

By the end of the night, I've lost about a quarter of my shiny new haircut.

Jack stands — having seen enough — and shuts down our hair-pulling party, looking slightly sick to his stomach.

"Goodnight, everybody," he announces, opening the front door.

After our guests take their exit cue, he escorts me up the stairs to bed.

"That was weird," he states.

"Oh come on," I defend my friends' dark humor. "It was all in good fun. Do you want to grab a handful? It's fascinating."

"Deirdre, sometimes …"

"What?!"

"Some things are just not funny," he continues. "Like pulling out your hair by the handful. You know what it is?"

"What?"

"It's gross," he says, rolling away from me in bed. "Goodnight."

CHAPTER 13

Smooth move

Remember how I told you that they put me on steroids to keep my brain from swelling? Well, they're wreaking havoc on my perfect cancer figure and turning me into an eating machine. No amount of food can quell my hunger.

For breakfast, I snarf down bagels and eggs and bacon and granola.

When friends pick me up to take me to appointments, we stop for lunch on the way. I consume appetizers, entrees and desserts with abandon, sometimes ordering a second meal to eat in the car on the way to whatever appointment is next. I watch the clock like a hawk come dinnertime, waiting to light on the next meal train delivery like an eagle to a mouse. I have no shame dipping an entire chocolate bar into a jar of Jif and downing it like an anaconda swallowing an elk whole.

I grow out of my cancer clothes and back into my old wardrobe, lamenting my expansion as I handle up on breakfast burritos from Taco Time — utterly abandoning my cancer-killing diet of chard and garlic smoothies.

I turn into a mama lion pulling in her prey and baring her fangs when Jack says, "That's not on your diet! You're not supposed to eat that. You're killing yourself."

"At least I'll die happy," I tell him, narrowing my eyes. "Shove off."

But now, the joke's on me. After stuffing my gullet like a force-fed goose, all of that food has nowhere to go.

I cannot. Take. A shit.

Zofran, the anti-nausea medication — coupled with the steroids — have my bowels locked down tighter than Fort Knox.

I rummage through my medications. I realize they already have me on Sennecot and Ducolax. I was taking them completely unaware as to why. Well, cat's out of the bag, and these drugs are doing nothing, repeat NOTHING, to achieve any movement, shall we say.

As I'm finding in my journey through Candyland, Western nurses and techs and Eastern practitioners have the most valuable information in treatment-related symptoms (though nothing would save that hair, which is now almost completely gone). Doctors love to identify the root cause of the symptom and throw a pill at you, which opens the door to a whole new breed of unpleasant symptoms.

"Here," says one nurse administering my second round of chemo.

She gives me a constipation elimination handout entitled, "Gush, Push and Mush." Sound gross? It is, and I read it as if it contains the map to a pot of gold.

Drink lots of water. I do.

Take laxatives and stool softeners: I've doubled up on those.

Drink prune juice: Yes, I do.

It's been one week (SEVEN DAYS) since I've pooped and ain't none of this shit is helping. So I go to the Google, where I read to take magnesium (I start) and drink Smooth Move Tea, (Really? Couldn't they think of a better name?). When those don't work, I give myself an enema. That's a hell that I wouldn't inflict on my worst enemy. Not only is it awkward and painful to give yourself an enema, it does nothing.

Nothing.

Nada.

Rien.

Zilch.

Five days later and I'm starting to look pregnant. I now have 12 days of huge meals locked up inside me. I keep eating, because I'm famished thanks to the steroids. I don't get rid of anything in my gut because of all the reasons I just stated. And so I just swell and swell and swell. I can't bend at the waist, and I waddle like a duck.

"Maybe it's time for a colonic," Paula suggests.

Yes, a colonic! I think. Never before did the idea of having someone shove a tube up me arse and flush it with water sound so good. I fixate on getting a colonic.

I make an appointment at The Tummy Temple in Seattle's charming old neighborhood of Ravenna. Entering the incense-infused home that's been developed into a hair salon, and 'The Temple,' I'm practically giddy with anticipation to evacuate twelve days of poop.

The receptionist leads me to a small room where bland spa music plays, a table is draped by a wee-wee pad, a large machine with a tube sits against the back wall, and a toilet hides behind a curtain. As instructed, I remove my clothes from the waist down and climb onto the padded quasi-medical table, modestly covering my naked bottom with a thin blanket. There's a soft knock on the door and Heidi, my colonic savior, asks me to roll onto my left side and then, ever-so-gently, she shoves a tube up my butt.

"Oh! Hello!" I say. "OK. That just happened."

"Try to relax," Heidi recommends, like, maybe that advice will make this whole thing enjoyable.

"OK. I will just yes … try to relax," I say, squinting my eyes and clenching my teeth.

After pulsating the tube and flushing me with various "cleansing agents," Heidi gets … nothing.

"It's like concrete," she correctly notes.

"Yes, I know," I agree politely as she gets more aggressive pumping the tube up me arse.

People, I know this isn't ladylike talk, but this bitch is real and nobody really told me that I was soon going to embody the expression 'full of shit.' I was convinced that if I opened my mouth but barely, you'd see my last meal sitting at the back of my throat.

And then …

"Heidi!" I say, eyes wide in panic.

"Yes?" she calmly answers. She's a holistic practitioner and she smells like an aromatherapy parlor.

"I think I need to sit on the toilet … alone," I somewhat frantically tell her.

"OK," she says, rapidly pulling the tube from my nether regions. "Call me if you need anything."

I roll off the table and barely, I mean BARELY, sit on the pot in time to unleash weeks of grass-fed steaks, organic chickens, heirloom raspberries, blueberries and apples, and fucking chard smoothies. It's a purging that makes Mount St. Helens look like a drippy faucet. It is — quite literally — a shit show.

I flush.

I flush again.

I flush again and again and again.

"Everything OK in there?" Heidi yells through the door.

"Fine. Great," I yell back, lighting matches conveniently placed next to the toilet. "Don't come in here. The shit's going down and it's not pretty!"

After maybe twenty minutes of epic EPIC pooing something that looks (and smells) like a pungent cocktail of nuclear waste and rotten vegetables, I'm ready for a shower … and a well-earned nap.

Finally finished, I try to clean up as best I can and walk out of the room. As Heidi approaches me I warn, "Do NOT go in there!"

I leave The Tummy Temple one hour after entering — 10 pounds lighter, and 100 leagues happier.

No shit.

When I get home, I have a surge of energy, so I call Ada and cop a ride to Kathy's. I haven't seen her for three weeks, which is the longest I've gone without seeing her in years.

"Hi Mom, it's D-D, your daughter," I tell her, letting that introduction sink in before bending down to kiss her. "How are you?"

"Listen, I wanna go home," she says, looking through me.

"OK, I'll take you after lunch," I tell her. "You want to see my new hairdo?"

I take off my hat and present the biggest un-hairdo of all — basically a bald head with a few stray hangers-on.

"Oh, that's awful," she exclaims. "Why did you do that to your hair?"

"I didn't," I tell her. "I'm taking a medicine that made it fall out. Do you want to take this medicine?"

"Hell no," she says. "You look like Slitzy the Pinhead. Put your hat back on!"

Kathy's not in a good mood. Her arthritic hip pains her day in and day out. The staff have trained her to use a cane so she's steadier on her feet.

"This is nice," I say, pointing to the cane.

"What is it?" she asks.

"A cane, to help you walk."

"Fart and be damned, this is not fun!"

"What's not fun?" I ask.

"All … this," she says, pointing at the home's living room. "I want to go home."

CHAPTER 14

Did I die?

It's now mid-September and I have seven proton treatments and one chemo push to go before launching into nine daylong rounds of chemo infusions over the next nine months.

Rose has been in England for almost four weeks. During her travels, she's been regaling me with photos of her trip and Skyping me when she's near a computer. I don't want to dampen her fun, so I put my game face on and play down my own dark shadows, projecting that all is well in Candyland. For now, I want her to think radiation and chemo are a walk in the park and that our lives will go on together (even when I'm still not sure).

She'll be home during my last week of radiation. No longer scared that I would expose her to some damaging memories of her dying mother, I'm feeling pretty cocky that everything I'm doing in Candyland is killing Sara. Plus, I'm excited to show her the gantry and my ridiculous mostly-bald pate.

The tumor seems to be receding in the weekly MRIs, making me giddy with the prospect of finishing this portion of treatment and easing into nine months of heavy chemo to kill every last little popcorn scent of Sara.

I'm no longer dizzy as a bat, and though I'm very weak, it's with great relief that I can walk in a straight(ish) line. The constant stream of visitors has kept boredom at bay (not to mention my new best friend, TV). No longer able to swing two-mile walks, I struggle to walk the dogs to the end of our block and back. I need assistance to stand up or walk down stairs, and tasks as simple as rolling over in bed are challenging. But I know this weakness is temporary, and the dogs seem perfectly happy with short walks and spending the rest of the day on the couch with me.

In addition to Ada, my friend Susan from Chicago and my friend Mia from Portland travel to Seattle to maintain the house, do the shopping, and most thankfully, massage my head, which aches constantly as the hair follicles die.

My hair, eyelashes and eyebrows are mostly gone, (I have six eyelashes on my left eye, and four eyelashes on my right eye). Even though it's approaching late September, I wear hats to cover my distractingly sparse hair and keep my head warm. I have to pack on the face powder to hide the dark circles under my eyes caused by low blood cell counts. If I have to dress up, which is rare, I wear a wig that approximates my natural hair and paint on cat-eye makeup to mask the lack of eyelashes and draw on eyebrows so I don't look so obviously cancerous (though I do feel like a clown with all this frippery).

My cancer treatment fucks with my skin, my hair, my weight, my posture, my gait, my everything. I move like an old lady, grabbing handrails as if they're buoys in a storm, falling, and sometimes standing from a sitting position after several failed attempts. I consider using a walker when I just can't walk Arthur more than the distance of four houses.

As I struggle to get out of the car and wait for someone to take my arm, I use my free arm to adjust my slipping wig.

"Is my wig on straight?" I ask my escort *du jour*.

Then I chide my friends when they take my picture and my wig is riding way up on my head and I look like a drunken clown.

"Delete that, NOW," I tell them.

I only wear wigs when I'm going out and I just don't want to see all the *Ohhh, poor-thing-has-cancer* looks. But when I do wear wigs they still look funny because, well, they're made of plastic.

When I do manage to kind of look normal with makeup, fake hair, and a cute outfit, I'm buried under three layers of winter clothes even though it's midsummer and I have tennis shoes on because my balance is so bad and my feet hurt from chemo, which is causing nerve damage.

I'm not really the most vain person (though I'm admittedly neurotic about my weight), but, well, I don't want to look sick and ugly. I want to look like a healthy middle-aged woman.

That, however, is impossible during this time. Even when I'm faking it you can see that things are not right in the State of Denmark.

I always imagined if I did pass on early in life, I would at least embody the phrase "Live fast, die young, and leave a good-looking corpse." But if I go during this time, I will not leave a beautiful corpse. And in my own vanity, that pisses me off. After all, I am Kathy's daughter. Years of her psychologically grooming my physical insecurity have succeeded in making me believe that — as Billy Crystal said on "Saturday Night Live" — "It's better to look good than to feel good."

My most surprising new symptom is radiation burns. It hadn't occurred to me that these intense rays would burn me on the outside — I thought they were strictly scorching my insides. But no. My scalp is red and burned. My ears resemble pink cauliflower. My eyes are swollen and bloodshot. My forehead and neck are red and dry and red and dry and red and dry. And my back sports a burnt and blistered streak snaking down my spine. I slather my back and ears with Eucerin throughout the day and beg for coconut oil head massages from any willing person at night.

As I grapple with my evolving looks, family's there to take the piss out of my vanity.

"You look beautiful, honey," laughs Jack. "Pretty enough to be on the cover of Reptile magazine."

"Ha ha, very funny," I snort. "Jerk. Pretty enough to be on the cover of Reptile magazine," I mockingly imitate him.

Nevertheless, he's hit on something that's very real: In Candyland, that which doesn't kill you makes you uglier.

Even Kathy has fun with the balding and burns.

"You look like you've been et by a bear and shit off a cliff," she smirks, only half joking on my latest visit.

I've gained 15 pounds, thanks to the steroids. While I'm still thin, I'm no longer boney (which bums me out because I loved being boney thin). My constipation from steroids and anti-nausea medication persists. That's a bummer.

While all of my doctors tell me I'm doing well, I'm tired of the rigamarole. I want to have a normal poop. My scalp hurts. My feet ache and tingle from the effects of chemo on my nervous system. Add that to all of the pill popping and herb swilling and — while I know this is temporary — I feel like I'm going a little crazy. It's like being force-fed McDonald's Super Size meals when you've been a vegan your whole life. The steroids continue to make me eat like a football lineman and they keep me up all night, so I have to take Ambien to fall asleep — and then take another one when I wake up at 2 in the morning, hungry.

But as impatient as I am with all this, I am starting to feel cocky that I'm handling everything relatively well, so I devise a brilliant plan to wean myself off all my drugs so my body only has to deal with chemo and radiation.

After all, I was never nauseous, even though I took anti-nausea medication.

And I'm still a titch dizzy, even though I take steroids for dizziness.

And I have to take FIVE medications for constipation caused by the steroids and anti-nausea drugs, and I'm still constipated!

It's like, STOP THE INSANITY!

So, what do I do? I go renegade, shoving pills to the back of my cupboard, ignoring that they ever existed. I tell my doctor I'm doing it. She says she wouldn't do it, but she can't force me.

Riiiight.

In a matter of a few short days, I realize the Western cowboys have pretty much figured this gig out. They prescribe these drugs for a reason. About three days into my new drug-free existence, I don't want to leave my bed; I become dizzier (God, I can't wait for that to end); my appetite disappears (I not-so-secretly love that); and I want to throw up pretty much all the time.

So I do what any good chef would do and I jump back in the frying pan and go back on everything. And now I trust the drugs, even though I don't like them. And although they help, they can't fix everything. There are a few things I can no longer tolerate. According to my ultimate source for all things true, Mr. Wikipedia: "Aversion therapy is a form of psychological treatment in which the patient is exposed to a stimulus while simultaneously being subjected to some form of discomfort."

I'd say radiation counts as "some sort of discomfort" and is probably why I've developed some pretty strong associations in Candyland. Some of them, aversions.

Turmeric, which is apparently very good for antagonizing Sara, I now completely associate with Brain Candy and never want to eat again.

Garlic. Ditto.

Smoothies. Ditto (times a thousand).

Curry. Yup. Ditto.

Green tea. Nettle tea. Ginger tea. Licorice tea. Check. Check. Check. And check.

Carrots (which is odd, because I've barely eaten any, but they're always in my fridge, looking at me, just threatening that I will have to eat them).

Then there's music. I listened to Lana Del Ray on Pandora during my first couple of weeks of radiation. Sorry, Lana. I will always associate you with cancer now. And I loved you so much.

Things that I normally loved, I can't even fathom consuming now. Mainly, red meat and booze. Gah-what? They just taste wrong. Interestingly, Wikipedia says, "The major use of aversion therapy is currently for the treatment of addiction to alcohol." Hmmmm.

Oh, and the things that I will probably always associate with my time in WooWooVille that I hope to stick with for the rest of my life? My daily walks (looking forward to returning to my two-plus miles through forests and along the beach with a big hill-climb at the end). Herbs (I HATE HATE HATE taking pills, but I truly believe they're healthful). Acupuncture, which apparently balances my chi, (but all I know is it makes me feel gah-happy.) Massage (I've become a regular at Seattle's Chinese reflexology centers where you get a full massage for $30/hour). And perhaps a little Reiki now and then (can't really define how it seems to help. It just ... does).

As I sit watching the "Today" show and navel-gazing about my aversions, Jack hangs up the phone. I assume he's been talking to his project lead at the high-tech company he's working with.

"Knuckle me baby," says Jack, holding his fist out for a fist bomb. "Just got my first investor!"

"What?" I ask, bumping knuckles with him. "Are you kidding?"

"I wouldn't shit my favorite turd," he glows, pulling out a celebratory cigar. "Just 23 more investors and I can buy the property."

"Just 23?" I ask. "That sounds like a lot."

"The first one's the hardest one," he explains. "Now that I have one investor, others should start to jump on board."

"Alright, let's hope so. It sounds like you have your hands on the helm," I smile with pride. "Ships ahoy!"

For the last week of radiation, I decide to start going to my radiation appointments early. Over the past few weeks I've befriended many of the other patients who have appointments at the same time. There's Garrett, a 5-year old boy with a wicked sarcoma growing out of his eye. And Henry, who is battling cancer for the third time and is no longer walking. There's John, whose teenage son has to wear a brain bucket since his skull is open to relieve pressure from brain swell. There's another John, a young man with spinal cancer. He's very bitter about his cancer, and understandably so — a tumor wraps around the entire length of his spinal cord, and he is now paralyzed. There's a Mexican man who doesn't speak English, but he sits near our cancer klatch to vibe off our laughter and camaraderie.

"Check this out," I say to Jim, one of the other patients. I lift my shirt, turn my back toward him, and show him my burnt spine. "Impressive, no?"

"Oh, sweetie," he says. "I'm burnt too."

"Prove it," I joke. He has prostate cancer.

I deeply appreciate my new radiation friends.

Some things you just don't want to burden your family and friends with. Limping through the wearying fog of finality is not only intense, it's deeply personal and even a little shameful. I don't know why it's shameful. Maybe because it takes you out of the game of regular life and sets you in a completely different direction — a direction you didn't choose where nobody else can go unless they're in the same predicament.

And though my cancer buddies are virtual strangers, our situation brings us immediately close. We discuss our varying symptoms like it's top-secret business.

Steroids have made several of us awkwardly emotional, causing us to cry over the smallest details, like burnt toast or a leaky sink. We discuss the most intimate topics — how our spouses are responding to becoming unsolicited caregivers, the embarrassment of impotence during treatment, or in my case, a total lack of sexual desire.

We share feelings of guilt, guilt over becoming dysfunctional and downright disabled. We display raidation burns, discuss painful hands and feet, and talk about sleepless nights, constipation, fatigue, and confusion — symptoms we all suffer from. We indulge in our misery together, often laughing at the drama of Candyland.

But not all of us cave to the pity party in the radiation center lobby. Specifically, the children.

They run into the building, bald-headed and brave. They often make a beeline for the playroom while their exhausted and frightened parents sit apart from the adult cancer patients and try to hold it together.

Five-year-old Garrett's unbridled joy and complete disinterest in his very sobering situation has been perhaps one of the greatest gifts to me during this time. He doesn't feel sorry for himself. When he enters the center, he seems completely unaware of the sarcoma living on his right eye. He always bears a smile and is a bright ray of joy, filling the large room with his high voice, his child's energy, and his joyous laughter.

As we adults grumble and moan, Garrett shows us how to be a true soldier. His brazen optimism and momentous bravery are infectious and uplifting. Running alongside his parents and seemingly delighted to be here, Garrett embodies the wisdom of youth.

Garrett helps guide me — and everyone who swims in his wake at the proton center. He shows us to tread the Candyland pool with blue skies, sunshine, deep breaths, neon lollipops … and fearless fighting.

If he can be happy, so can we.

I'm even getting a little mournful that I'll be leaving my little ragtag team of survivors in a few short days. I feel as if we have been climbing Mount Everest together, delving into life, death, love lost, love gained, aspirations, hopes and fears. I find it so refreshing that the gravity of our situation has created a no-bullshit atmosphere, and probably for the first time in my life, I'm hearing men bare their souls and speak from the heart, even though we are strangers.

There's no candy-coated bullshit when we're together.

Since my weekends are mercifully free of any treatments I have enough energy to visit my mother. My dear friend Susan, who is visiting from Chicago for a couple of weeks to help us out (and gives me amazing two-hour head massages with coconut oil) takes me to see Kathy. Susan used to live across the street from my mother and has shared a complicated past with my mom. Long before we knew Kathy had Alzheimer's, she would say and do nonsensical things to Susan that were often, quite frankly, mean. Thankfully, Kathy doesn't remember her queer past with Susan, and Susan has kindly forgiven her, and now Kathy just adores Susan.

"Isn't she pretty?" Susan asks Kathy, pointing at me.

Today, I'm wearing a wig because I didn't want Kathy to cycle on my missing hair.

"She's beautiful," Kathy jokes. "She got it all from me."

Then, Kathy turns to me.

"Where's my dad?" she asks.

"He died about 40 years ago," I tell her.

"Did Fred [my dad] die?" she presses on.

"He died a year ago," I tell her.

"Did I die?" she asks.

"Not yet," I tell her, pulling out one of her old family albums to try to situate her.

"Who's that?" she asks, pointing at an old picture of a mustachioed man.

"That's my great great great Uncle Charlie," I tell her. "I think he looks like me."

"Nope," she looks at me. "He's much better looking."

"Alright, you win," I laugh. I really love how even though Mom's deeply steeped in her Alzheimer's, she can still pull punchline after punchline. She was a nurse all her life, but I always felt she missed her calling as a TV comedy writer.

"Who's that?" she asks, this time pointing to the TV.

"That's Mark Wright, the weather guy," I tell her.

"He's kinda cute," she notes. "But he's not my type. My type is dead."

🌀 🌀 🌀

You know how you never hear about a thing — until that thing is part of your life — and then you hear about that thing constantly?

Well, that's me 'n' Brain Candy.

"What did you do yesterday?" I asked a friend this week.

"I went to the most amazing funeral," she said. "The woman was only 33, but she was so cool and so loved."

"Oh, I'm sorry. What did she die of?" I asked.

"Brain cancer."

Ribbet.

I have avoided researching my situation. I find cancer books with stories of success bring me up, only to drop me like a ton of bricks with stories of failed treatment. I basically just want to remain ignorant, as if what I don't know won't kill me. I let Jack and Don and Ada carry the weight of tracking exactly what's going on during my protocol. By ignoring all information, I feel like I'm not letting the disease seep into my psyche and dicker with my chances of survival.

Though my first oncologist quoted a 60 percent chance of survival, none of my other doctors have quoted that statistic. So I wonder: *Was he correct or just trying to be encouraging?* Don knows. When he began reading up on my situation, he asked me if I wanted to know.

"No," I told him, choking on the thought of my imminent demise. "It's just too scary."

"Do you want to know your cure rate?" my chemo oncologist asked me a week ago.

"No," I tell him. "It's just too scary."

Jack and I don't discuss my survival either. I don't want to. He doesn't want to. I'm just more comfortable talking about it with my cancer buddies. He's distracted by and excited about his restaurant. I sense he's tired of cancer talk. These days we reserve our conversations to his restaurant fund-raising and Rose's travels and the weather and — anything but *What if?*

But now, with radiation ending soon and Rosie returning from England in a few days, I'm ready to know.

When I get home, I finally research the question that nobody dares ask, including myself.

What are my real chances of survival? Or, in Wild West lingo, what is my "cure rate"?

Is Deirdre dying, or is she just a drama queen doing time in Candyland?

I open my laptop, and hit GOOGLE.

Bring it on, I say to myself, running my hand through Arthur's mane, then placing my hands on the keyboard.

And this is what I find.

The most recent data show that 60 percent of adults with medulloblastoma have a five-year survival rate. This does not include factors in my favor (no metastasis at time of diagnosis, more modern treatment, favorable subtype), all of which lower my risks. And, it does not mean if I am in the 60 percent success rate, I am limited to only five more years on this Earth. That's just how long they've tracked that group of survivors in the most recent studies.

My *first* oncologist was right!

Oh my God, I sigh to myself. This thing that I've been pretending doesn't matter and that I've been psyching myself into believing it will not kill me — probably won't. I'll be OK. I got this one — I really, honestly, probably do got this one.

A weight I hadn't even realized was crushing my soul, lifts.

I don't know if confirming my encouraging chances of survival on WebMD does it or what, but at this very moment I look out of my window and realize — for the first time in two years — I'm not dizzy.

I put my laptop down and stand up. OK, it's still a struggle to stand and I still snake my way to my desk, but I pull out a pen and paper and guess what? I can write!!! It's been weeks since I've been able to scratch out a sentence or even sign my name, and even though the sentence I print — "Can Deirdre write?" — is barely legible, the words are legible and the sentence is clear.

I look at the sentence,: "Can Deirdre write?" I look around the living room. It's stable.

Did confirming my chances of survival change things? I wonder. *Or at that very moment was treatment starting to work?*

With tears streaming down my face, I look at Arthur.

"I'm gonna live sweetie," I tell him. He cocks his head at an angle trying to understand if this sudden burst of emotion means he's getting a treat.

BARK. BARK! BARK! He blasts.

"Yeah, OK," I shush him, standing to retrieve a doggie treat. "We're gonna have to start walking a lot more! You're my personal trainer, Arthur. We're gonna walk every day. We'll start by going around the block tomorrow. You need to help me get stronger 'cuz Mama ain't goin' nowhere!"

CHAPTER 15

Graduation

I haven't been able to make it to Kathy's since my last visit more than a week ago. This makes me feel sooooo guilty.

Whether or not it's true, I view my role as not only her loving daughter, but as her Rock of Gibraltar. There is no way I will be able to get to her as I wrap up this round of treatment.

"Bonnie," I say into the phone. "It's Deirdre."

"Deirdre, how are you?" asks the cheerful receptionist at my mom's home.

"Good, actually, I mean, considering," I tell her. I really don't know what 'good' means anymore. "I finish radiation this week and Rose will be home soon."

"That's great!" she says. "When will we see you next? We miss you."

"I know. That's what I'm calling about," I say. "How's my mom? I miss her."

"We have her using a walker now because her bad hip has made her pretty unstable. But she's learning to use it really well."

"Oh, good," I say, picturing my once strong and unstoppable mother humping along with a walker. "Will you give her a hug for me? And I'll come by the first day I can."

"Sure Deirdre," she assures me. "You don't need to worry about your mom. She's doing fine."

Bonnie's words wrap around me like a warm blanket, and I exhale in relief.

"Jump up," I command Arthur after hanging up the phone. "Let's take a walk and see if we can walk around the block!"

Rosie returns from her adventures in England today. She left four weeks ago when I was just beginning radiation. The last time she saw me, I was still in a state of shock over my diagnosis. Hell, we all were.

Though I've spent most of my time swaddled on the couch with my furry friend Arthur, it seems that so much has happened during her monthlong absence. I swung from fear of imminent death to belief that I would kick this somber disease. As opposed to planning my funeral and writing my obit, which is basically where I was when she left, I've started allowing myself to daydream about her high school graduation, her future career, her possible marriage, and best of all, her future motherhood.

When Jack's car pulls into the driveway, I start panting. I watch as my six-foot tall gazelle gracefully steps out of the car and looks toward the window, waving when she sees me. I try to wave in return, but as I hold my hand up, I freeze, except for the tears streaming down my face.

When the front door opens, I can't move.

"Oh, Mama," Rose says, coming over to me and hugging me. "Don't cry."

"Oh, baby," I blubber. "I didn't know if I was ever gonna see you again."

Now she's crying. "But you did. Here I am."

We remain locked in embrace, not saying anything.

"Your baby's home," Jack says, walking through the door with her luggage.

"I know," I say, still crying. "Promise me you'll never leave again."

"I can't promise that, Mama," she smiles.

"I know," I tell her. "Just lie. Lie for me."

"OK…" she humors me. "I promise I will never leave this house ever again."

"Good," I say, pulling her closer to me.

With Rose in the house, life seems soft, serene and comfortable. I'd been so distracted since my diagnosis that I hadn't realized how much I missed her. She spends the next few weeks baking goodies, perfuming the house with molten chocolate and special teas that she brought back from England. Perhaps a little shocked at how weak I am, she volunteers to do the laundry (!) and walk the dogs (!!). Jack also breathes a sigh of relief that she is here to share the emotional burden of our current reality.

I know it could be a pipe dream, but I'm hoping to have my final radiation treatment next Friday and then hop on a plane to attend my dear friend Julyne's wedding in New York this weekend. It's going to be tough considering my exhaustion, my compromised immune system and my frail state, not to mention I haven't purchased my airline ticket because my inner voice is screaming, "Deirdre, you can't finish radiation on Friday, then fly to the East Coast and just start celebrating like a rock star!"

"Do you think you'll be able to come?" Julyne asks when I'm on the phone with her. Julyne and I met 15 years ago at a journalism conference and we've been great friends ever since. Though she moved to New York more than six years ago, our friendship has remained resolute thanks to cell phones and Facebook and regular visits. "It's in less than a week, honey. I have a room for you and everything. You won't have to do anything. I just want you to walk down the aisle with me."

"Yes," I hesitate. "But the timing will be tight. And I'm weak, you know. I don't want to be a burden."

"You wouldn't be a burden," she appeals. "I love my Deirdre. I want you there."

We hang up with no definitive resolution.

I don't want to let Julyne down by not coming, but I don't want to bring her down by coming. And then, fate steps in. Remember the gantry? It's the radiation cannon that has been shooting me silly for the past five weeks. Three days before the wedding, I'm lying locked into my body case and head mask. After many stops and starts, engineers enter and leave my radioactive womb.

"We have to reset the gantry, Deirdre," says a voice on the loudspeaker. "Sit tight."

Hours, days, weeks seem to pass. Every bone in my body aches from immobility due to my complete confinement. My teeth feel like they're going to fall out from the tight pressure of my mask. I begin to sweat and panic from claustrophobia.

"How much longer?" I manage to mumble with the vice grip restricting my mouth.

"Just a few more minutes," the encouraging voice tells me.

This. Is. Hell.

Then, the gantry heaves one last deep sigh and shuts down.

"OK Deirdre, we're done for today," says the voice.

The techs remove the mask and pull my legs and arms loose from the body cast, hoisting my aching body into a sitting position.

"What was that all about?" I ask, pissed that I was in the gantry for so long.

"The gantry is broken," says the tech.

"Jesus, how long was I in there?" I ask, exhausted and sore.

"Four and a half hours," says Nikki. "I didn't tell you because we thought we could fix it and complete this session."

"God damn, that was awful," I exclaim.

"I know," she apologizes. "But don't worry, the engineers and physicists can get it working by tomorrow. It'll set your treatment back a day, but you'll be able to finish on Monday."

"I have a wedding on the East Coast this weekend," I tell her.

"Yeah, you'll have to cancel," she says, gritting her teeth in an apologetic smile. "I'm really sorry."

So no wedding for me.

I know this sounds pedestrian, but it's the one wedding in my life I want to attend (well, besides Rosemary's). My friend Julyne has been yearning to find the right guy for 20 years, and when she finally did and it was apparent I was going to be alive, I planned on being there to share in her great joy. All of a sudden, I'm fed up.

Fed up with treatment.

Fed up with deferred life.

Fed up with cancer.

I get home full of piss and vinegar and cursing the gods (God? Yahweh? Allah? Buddha? Who cares? Not me now!). I feel like I'm abandoning a sister.

I get home and tell Rosemary and Jack, peppering my exclamation with many expletives.

"Why don't you send Rose in your stead?" asks Jack. "She's known Julyne all her life. She can represent."

"But I want to go," I whine like a child demanding a trip to Disneyland.

"But you can't go," he gently says.

"Yes I can," I start to spin. "I'll fly in Friday night to JFK, take a cab to the Queens Airport Connection, walk to the bus that goes to Green Port on Long Island, take a ferry to Shelter Island, and Julyne will pick me up." I'm starting to sound crazy and even I know in my weakened condition how preposterous this notion is. "I'll miss the rehearsal dinner but then I'll make it to the wedding. Then on Sunday I'll just, yeah, take a cab to the ferry, a bus to Long Island, and a cab back to the airport. I'll also miss the brunch, but by God I can go to the wedding and get back in time for my last radiation blast."

"You're getting hysterical," Jack tries to reason with me.

I look at him, eyes burning into his soul. Just when I think a forked tongue is going to unfurl from my mouth and wrap around Jack's neck and choke him, Rosemary intervenes.

"I'll go, Mama," she says, perfectly calmly. "I'll go for you."

My cheeks are hot. For some reason, this blip in the plan is really pissing me off. I'm madder about missing a wedding than having to slay Sara. I just had it in my head that I'd finish this fucking radiation and hop on a plane toasting champagne and basking in the glory of days without rays.

"I'd be happy to go," Rose reiterates.

I look from Rose to Jack to Rose, feeling like a cornered fox.

"It'll be good," she says, ever so sweetly. "I'll take lots of pictures."

And then I burst out crying.

"I really want to go," I say, sobbing like a child.

"I know, Mama," Rose says, hugging me in a motherly embrace. "Maybe Julyne's marriage won't last and you can go to the next one."

"Yeah," I sniffle. "That would be nice."

As Jack and Rose get ready to leave for the airport, I think of how my daughter's heading out to live my life for me. She will string lights, fluff hair, drink champagne, and carry peonies ... on my behalf. If I go, that will happen all the time. Rose will become my stand-in. I wave to Rose from the front door as Jack tosses her suitcase into the car and they back out of the driveway. I turn and look at the lilies that someone gave me on my dining room table. Lilies are the totem flower at funerals. I toss the lilies into the compost bin.

As I pout on my couch, the wedding party sends me texts of flowers, friends and speeches. Each one is like a blow to my heart. As one who's never been a fan of weddings, I don't quite understand why this is piercing my spirit. Maybe because it's such a palpable reminder of the kind of joys in life that I will not see if the protocol doesn't take and I slip away.

During the toasts, Julyne had told me she was going to have a moment of silence to acknowledge my absence.

"I'm not dead yet," I exclaimed, "but I wouldn't mind if you had a moment of laughter during the party to 'include' me."

"Done," said Julyne.

The wedding goes off without my divine presence and I see with hurtful clarity that I'm actually not necessary. Rose looks beautiful with the other bridesmaids, Julyne is ecstatic, and her fresh love is sealed. Julyne sends me a video of her toasting me at the wedding and thanking Rose for standing in for me, and it just wrecks me. With each new report, I open my cell phone and eat up the updates, crying harder with each one.

Still seething that I missed the wedding, Rose (who flew back on Sunday), volunteers to join me on wait for it ... wait for it ... THE LAST DAY OF RADIATION! That's right kids! This is it! The end of my first stage of treatment — radiation and chemo pushes. After tomorrow, there will be no more sadistic strap-downs and my burnt scalp, ears, eyes and spine can start to heal. Though I adore the crew at the proton treatment and I will miss my cancer klatsch with other patients, I feel like an Olympic athlete nearing the finish line of the first leg of a race. After this, I'll just have monthly infusions for the next nine months.

I've made good on a promise to Garrett that I'd play dress-up during our last few treatments. Garrett, my 5-year-old shaman and radiation comrade continues to be a beacon in the storm thanks to his uber happy attitude and his complete disregard for the threat on his life. On Thursday, I dress as Marie Antoinette in a marshmallow of a wig. On Friday, I glam it up a là Lady Gaga with long platinum hair and a strapless cheetah dress. Rose pulls out her extensive makeup collection and helps me primp for my role as a '50s mom, with an electric pink bobbed wig and cat-eye makeup.

When we enter the center, all the patients cheer and clap — partially because the costume is so fun, but mostly because this is my last day of radiation. Before heading into my final session, I hug each patient goodbye. Most of them I'll never see again, unless they are at the graduation party that ProCure hosts for patients finishing radiation. Their sessions are much shorter than mine and they'll be out the door before I finish. With each hug, we bid each other good luck and thank one another for the tenderness that we've shared.

Since a living creature can only take so much nuclear blasting before growing a second head, when you leave ProCure, it will be the last time you walk through those doors. It's kind of a once-in-a-lifetime opportunity. And so ProCure hosts an actual graduation party for patients when they're finished because it's a big accomplishment; it costs a bloody fortune (my insurance is still haggling with us over who should pay for the radiation); and it's like graduating high school, once you walk out those doors, you ain't never coming back.

Guy — a Desert Storm vet, ProCure's head of operations, and a teddy bear of a man — delivers a tear-filled speech about the battles we fight. Now, we all fight battles. I have my current very obvious one. But you reading this … you have yours. Your loved ones have theirs. Your enemies have theirs. We all have them. Some we win. Some we lose. Some just fizzle out.

But for me, this graduation represents one battle down in a much grander war of fighting for life. As I scan the room of staff, cancer patients, family and friends, tears roll down my cheeks. I feel a deep affection for my cancer comrades. Swords drawn, this small group of friends and I have been peering into the eye of the dragon. As the beast belched fire from its gaping maw, we struck back. I'll miss our raw discussions about our fatigue, our loved ones, our appetites, our mental fog, the uncertainty of life, the weather — and discussing other stuff too, the Oprah stuff — like how we NEVER take a day for granted now, or how much love we've found in the world that was there all along but we never really saw it, or just how totally connected we all are to each other simply because, like war veterens we've fought the same battle at the same time.

The morning of graduation, I don my favorite blue dress and wake up Rose, insisting she come. Jack too has been badgered into putting on a suit and waiting for his preening girls.

We enter the proton center's large elegant lobby. My family gravitates to the catered lunch while I make the rounds, laughing with techs and doctors and staff and the other graduates. I feel so close to them all.

So as Renee, ProCure Hostess With The Mostess, calls out the graduates' names and hands us our medals (I'm number 47) and our "degrees," it is with overwhelming emotion that I smile at my family, hug Renee and truly feel like this might be the most important graduation of my life.

CHAPTER 16

Lick it

Candyland is like a funhouse of clichés: That which doesn't kill you makes you stronger. When life gives you lemons, make lemonade. Today is the first day of the rest of your life. Here today, gone tomorrow ....

And as you maneuver distorted rooms and swinging bridges, you just want to get out of there and return to straight walls, still paths and a clean bill of health.

Not only do I start my chemo regime today, but we get to see what Sara's up to in the house of clichés — is she growing like a leaf or is she dead as a doornail?

"How do you feel?" my chemo oncologist asks.

"I don't feel like a drunken sailor anymore, so that's promising," I tell him. "But my feet hurt a lot and my hands are going numb."

"That's the Vincristine," he says, typing on the computer. "We'll remove it from your next round of chemo."

"Don't I need it?" I ask, thinking that was just too easy.

"Your body's not reacting well to it. I'll just replace it with Lomustine, which is easier on your blood," he explains. "Is there anything else?"

"I'm really weak and tired," I tell him.

"Exercise," he tells me. "It seems counterintuitive to exercise when you're weak and tired, but it's the only way to gain strength and energy."

"Actually, I can barely walk," I tell him, more than a little irked by his seeming insouciance.

"Swim," he suggests. "Anything else?"

Unlike my massage therapist and my acupuncturist and the reiki practitioners and my friends bringing meal train and get-well cards, this doctor is all business. His matter-of-fact carriage makes me feel like an engineering project, not a human.

"Yeah, there is something else," I tell him. "I still can't poop. CANNOT poop."

"Double up on your Senecot and Ducolax," he suggests.

"I already did," I tell him.

"Well, again, exercise will help with that," he tells me.

"But, again, I'm really weak and tired. Plus, I'm still a total spaz when I try to do anything. My right and left side are just not in sync. And my right side is completely floppy."

"Touch my finger then touch your nose with your left hand," he instructs, launching into the battery of exercises he has me do to see how my left and right sides are performing. "Now do it with your right hand. Now follow my finger with your eyes. Good. Come out in the hallway with me. I want to see you walk."

"You look great," he observes. "I'm not seeing any compromised movement."

"OK, I'm not dizzy, but I'm not right either. I'm off-kilter," I try to explain. I want him to produce some magic bullet to stop the symptoms of the tumor and the treatment, but apparently he's not packing any heat.

"Is the latest MRI in?" Jack asks, shifting this frustrating conversation.

The MRI! I forgot about the MRI. That's why we're here — to see if the tumor is gone! This will be the first time we've seen my brain since I began radiation.

"It is," he says turning to his computer and pulling up the scans. "The tumor is still there, though it will probably be there the rest of Deirdre's life."

"What?" I ask. "What do you mean, 'It will probably be there the rest of Deirdre's life'"?!

"The brain does not slough cells like the rest of the body," he continues his cruel diatribe. "So you will probably have the tumor the rest of your life, but what we're hoping is that it's dead."

"You mean, I'm not cured?" I ask, holding back tears. "What if one cell is still alive and what if it … reanimates?"

"That's a possibility," he candidly says.

FUCK! I wanted to walk out of this appointment dancing a jig and screaming out, "I'M CANCER FREE, BITCHES!!!!"

"Won't the chemo kill it?" I ask, sinking into a massive dose of disappointment.

"Chemo doesn't cross the bloodbrain barrier," he says.

"Then why are we doing it?" Jack steps in.

"In case the cancer has spread," says the doctor, shifting his attention back to Jack. "You have to remember, Deirdre had a grade 4 tumor. It was fast-growing. But, if we compare this MRI to her first one before radiation, we can see that the tumor has reduced in size and it is no longer pushing against the rest of her brain. That's great news. Tumors don't tend to get smaller if they're alive."

"So it's dead?" Jack makes him reiterate that piece of information.

"It's inconclusive," the doctor says, explaining that Sara is like a dead body in my brain that the brain has yet to consume and a single surviving cancer cell can start the growth all over again. "For now, it looks good."

"For now?" Jack asks. "What do you think are the chances it will reanimate?"

"There's no way to know that," he says, matter-of-factly. "We'll take MRIs every couple of months and hope for the best. After a year, if we can't detect any new growth in the tumor, we reduce to an MRI every six months. If we still see no growth in a year, then we reduce her MRIs again to once a year. After three years of annual MRIs and if — again — there is no change, we'll assume the tumor is dead. That will be five years after Deirdre was first diagnosed and with no changes in her X-rays, Deirdre will be considered cancer-free."

I knew from my reading that five years was considered the magic number — if there are no new tumors or if my current tumor doesn't grow — then I would be considered "cancer free." But somehow, hearing this now, I feel like this is going to be a five-year game of holding my breath and playing the lottery of life.

"Meanwhile," continues my doctor, "let's get you started on the next round of chemo."

"OK, I guess," I tell him, thoroughly disappointed that none of my symptoms have been addressed and Sara has only lost a little weight but she's still at the party.

As Jack and I wend our way through the hospital maze to leave, Jack is silent.

"Well, that was fun," I say. "Five years of waiting, worrying and wondering."

"I'm sorry, honey," he says, taking my arm. "It sucks."

"Tcha! It really sucks."

I look down the long hallway. Again with the tears. I've never been a crier, and I'm seriously beginning to resent my growing penchant for uncontrollable tears. This whole thing is getting less and less funny. Not that it was ever funny, but I'm losing sight of my humor and my ability to use laughter as my strongest coping mechanism.

After my disheartening oncologist appointment, I need a Kathy visit. Seeing her is so comforting, even though she generally has no idea who I am and where we are. Still, I know how to make her smile and every chuckle I get out of her is like a spoonful of feel-good medicine for me. With Kathy, black humor is totally acceptable. I can spill my guts to her. We can cry. We can then switch to silliness. And she can swing with whatever feelings I need to work through, granting me full freedom to have crazy manic blowouts over the whole goddamned trauma. And when I leave, she won't be taxed by my breakdowns because she won't remember a thing.

"What happened here?" she asks, pointing at my bald head. Again.

"I had brain cancer and they gave me a medicine to cure it, but the medicine made my hair fall out," I explain. Again.

"Oh, God in Heaven, why did you do this to my little girl?" she asks, looking up to the ceiling. I'm so happy she remembered that I'm her daughter.

"It's OK Mom, I'm cured," I lie. "It just left me looking like a plucked chicken."

"We've had terrible things happen to our family," says Kathy.

"Like what?" I ask.

"Well, my two sisters both lost their feet," she continues. "So they got feet from other people that didn't need them anymore."

"Which sisters were they?" I ask.

"The little ones about three feet tall," she tells me.

"Oh my," I say. Kathy is really in a strange place.

"Your father has been giving me a fair trial," she switches gears.

"How so?" I ask, not bothering to remind her that my dad has been dead for more than a year.

"He gets sicker and sicker and doesn't want to eat and doesn't want to drink."

"Hmmm," I tell her. "He is a stubborn one."

"Ya got that right," she says, holding her arthritic hand up and inspecting it. "That hurts."

"What hurts? I ask.

"Right there, I burned this finger," she explains.

"How'd you burn it?" I ask.

"Baking," she explains.

I've never known my mother to bake in her life. "What did you bake?"

"Chocolate pumpkin," she answers.

"Mmmm," I say. "It's been a long time since I've had chocolate pumpkin. What is chocolate pumpkin, Mom?"

And then we both bust out in laughter.

"Hell I don't know, but I made it," she chuckles.

Ahhhh, that's what I needed. Just a shade of the ridiculous with one of the greatest loves of my life.

My oncologist decides to give my body some time to recuperate from the toxic blasting it's just endured, so I have a month off before the hard-core chemo begins.

I welcome the break from machines, hospital gowns, fluorescent lights and needles.

I am weaker and more tired than I have been throughout this whole adventure, but one of the radiation nurses explains that's to be expected as my body has now completed a major assault and it's deeply wounded.

"Be patient," the doctor explains. "With time you will recuperate. This is probably the worst you'll feel during all of treatment. Your body is processing the culmination of six weeks of radiation and chemo."

At the end of the month off, I still feel weak and exhausted, but today I'm scheduled for my first daylong chemo infusion. At the peak of my malaise — I rise early, I shower, and Ada drives me to UW Medical Center. First, I must have my blood drawn to make sure it is strong enough to receive my new chemo cocktail of Cisplatin and Lomustine. I don the all-too-familiar toothpaste-green gown, then I'm shown to a private cubby on the chemo ward, complete with a bed, heavenly warm blankets, a TV, and a fantastic view of the Montlake Cut in the University District. I sip my brown rice tea, waiting for the lab to send my blood results to the ward.

"Good news," my oncology nurse steps in, taking my vitals before inserting my IV. "You're good to go. Your chemo has been ordered and should be here shortly. In the meantime, we're going to start hydrating you with a Saline drip."

"Oh goodie goodie," I tell her.

My hair has started to grow back and I have what looks like a very hip hairstyle a la Sinead O'Connor in the '80s.

"Look," I tell the nurse, extremely proud of my shadow of growth. "I was told my hair would never grow back after radiation, and ha-ha, it's growing back!"

"Nice," she says, "but don't get too attached to it because it's going to start falling out again."

Ahhhhh, shit, I think to myself. *I knew it was too good to be true.*

Another nurse hands her a large clear plastic bag boldly marked **CHEMO**.

"That must be mine," I say breezily. "Let the party begin."

The nurse pulls on her hazmat gear, because remember, this is so poisonous that even a drop on her skin could cause damage. The very same poison that's getting pumped into my veins. Yup.

My saline bag is almost empty, so she detaches it and replaces the IV feed with a cocktail of 10 mg Decadrone (steroids), a dash of Zofran (for anti-nausea), and 130 mg of Cisplatin (chemo).

"OK, Deirdre, this will take six hours or so to be absorbed. When it's finished we'll give you another bag of saline solution for added hydration. Then I'll send you to the pharmacy in the basement where they'll give you Lomustine in a pill. You'll have to take it in front of the pharmacist," she says, tossing her hazmat suit and goggles into the hazmat trash. "Here is your call button. Just buzz if you need anything. If you want to order food or a drink, here is the menu. The food's pretty good here. Do you want to watch TV?"

Knowing I would be here all day, I have planned the shows I want to watch: the "Today" show to catch up on humanity's frivolity; "I Dream of Genie" to revisit a time in my life when I believed a buxom blond could live in a bottle; "Ellen" to laugh. I also brought my computer and my cell phone, predicting that I would turn them off to sleep.

I've instructed all of my family and friends that I do not want visitors while receiving chemo — I want to rest without having to make small talk.

My house has been a train station of friends and family dropping by at all hours. Don't get me wrong, I LOVE the company, but being present for people as they flow in and out the front door is exhausting. My situation brings up so many issues for people and what they've experienced with illness or lost loved ones, that I often feel like I'm playing the therapist listening to their stories and offering simple thoughts on finding peace within the great trial of life.

Since our culture is so predicated on "survival of the fittest," there are scant opportunities to ruminate on our dark uglies. But I now embody a dark ugly, and that struggle seems to provide a safe stage for people to share their struggles. My visitors climb under my blankets on the couch, sitting knee-to-knee with me, whispering their illnesses and tragic pasts, presumably because I am (hopefully) at my lowest stage in life and I cannot judge. Tales of lost loved ones, humiliating failures and unbearable challenges reverberate in my living room as I just keep my hand on their knee and nod my head in empathy.

As depleting as this new role can be, I like it. I like it as people share their genuine hopes and intimate fears. I like the soft-spoken honesty shared over coffee and pastries. I like walking through the forest of life hand-in-hand with people, our eyes and our hearts wide open (and our mobile phones silenced!). There's a sweetness to contemplating the question, "What is all this?" As my friends and I embrace a deeper shared experience — the seeds of our friendships feel like they're blooming into celestial gardens.

Eventually, these conversations hit 'the apology point.'

"I'm sorry, this must seem so mundane," they say. "I mean, how can I complain about my boyfriend TO YOU? Look what you're going through!"

"It's all good," I tell them. "It's nice to take a break from my mental looping and step onto somebody else's ride for a while. Good or bad. So, go on …"

Relieved at the permission to bitch and complain, they carry on.

However, just as having cancer has given me a break from the stress of my life, it feels like chemo sessions give me a break from the heady confessions that overwhelm my conversations of late.

I nestle into my hospital bed covered in heated blankets and surrounded by extra pillows I've requested, pondering this strange and amazing journey, as I watch the chemo drip into my veins. I marvel at the beauty outside my chemo cubby window and digest the kind swaddling of my family and friends during this chapter of my life.

Then I fall into slumber, relishing a day free of social obligation.

When my drip is finished, the nurse arrives to remove my IV and wake me.

"Is anyone picking you up?" she asks, as Jack pulls aside the curtain and enters my chemo cubby.

"I am," he says.

"Oh! I didn't know you were there!" she jumps. "Deirdre did very well today. She'll need to rest and make sure she drinks a lot of water tonight."

"Got it," he says.

Although I feel swollen from the steroids and plucked bald from the chemo, Jack remembers to look in my eyes and say, "I love you." Twenty-five years of marriage dulled our attention to romantic detail and affection. We fell out of practice years ago from the simple acts of stopping, hugging, and saying those three simple words. Now, Jack watches me and sees me, really SEES me, looking into my eyes and tending to my needs — be they a foot rub, refilling my water glass, handing me my pills, or regaling me with his daily adventures.

During the past several months, Jack's been reeling in a growing number of investors for his future restaurant. While he still has a way to go, his daydream of opening Jack's BBQ edges ever closer to a reality.

"You'll have to help me design it," he smiles once we're home. "I'm thinking it should be like a genuine Texas 'cue joint, you know, casual and friendly."

"OK, honey," I share in his excitement. "I'll help you in whatever way I can."

"Hot damn," he says, shaking his martini shaker. "We're gonna have a restaurant! I can just feel it."

Rose is also excited. She starts her high school senior year in a few days and she has launched an earnest search for her next big step — college.

While she began her teenage detachment from me at 13 when she called a moratorium on physical affection of any sort — rendering kisses, hugs, snugglefests and hand-holding *verboten* — she has abandoned her Mommy divorce. She now — unsolicited — sits with me and cuddles on the couch, hugging and holding my hand and even letting me (gasp) kiss her on the cheek from time to time. Thanks cancer!

Arthur has also settled quite comfortably into their new docile lifestyle. They never harangue me as their walks shorten, patiently sleeping by my side while I run my fingers through their soft fur. Our neighbors' cat has adopted us, going home less and less and meowing at our back door more and more.

"Do you want your cat back?" I ask Regan, my neighbor.

"Well, yes, but he's chosen you," she generously notes. "You know, he's a cancer cat."

"What does that mean?" I ask her.

"His previous owner died of cancer," she explains.

"Wow," is all I have to say. This cat knew I had cancer and he came to offer comfort.

With no appointments for another month, family dreams on full throttle, and a new feline member in the house, the scent of a lively future perfumes our days with hope, affection and excitement.

After my first infusion, the vein that hosted my chemo IV turns red and swells with small hard balls like BBs forming in the vein. I email my doctor to let him know this is happening. If it doesn't resolve by the next chemo, he tells me, I can get a port.

A port, if you don't know, is a quarter-sized implant that is inserted subcutaneously into the left or right side of your upper chest with a line that funnels the chemo directly into your heart. With infusions as toxic as chemo, many patients opt for a port since the poison is fed directly into its destination and you don't risk damaging your veins. But I am vain (vein, argh), and I don't covet the thought of a port scar lingering in the corner of my décolletage, so I have opted to try the IV drip in my arms first.

"How are you, Deirdre?" asks my acupuncturist, David, who is now seeing me twice a week because my energy is severely flagging. David, who has also battled cancer, is one of the few people I feel comfortable going hatless or wigless around.

"Still can't poop," I tell him, comforted by his serene presence and his own experience with cancer. I know I can whine to him and he will have just the right soothing words I need to hear. "Still getting colonics. Feet still hurting. Still uncoordinated. Oh, and I'm getting seriously stupid. I mean, I can't remember anything anymore. I can't follow my calendar and I miss half of my appointments. Still freezing cold all the time. Still can't drive. Still tired — in fact more so than ever."

"Your body has taken an incredible beating," he notes. "Has anything good been happening with treatment?"

"Oh, right!" I respond, remembering that I have to cling to my silver linings. "I'm no longer as dizzy because Sara is no longer pushing against my brain. And that is what's most important."

"Deirdre, this is not an easy journey you're on," he reiterates. "But you've been handling all of this very admirably."

"That's because I rock," I joke with him. "Oh, and look at this new little nightmare. My vein is responding to the chemo and she is not happy. My doctor said to watch it and if it worsens we'll have to do something like cut off my arm and insert a port."

"Let's have a look at that," David says, gently taking my arm. He places my arm back on my lap. "I'm going to suggest something that may seem unorthodox."

"Shoot," I tell him. I love his crazy advice, like when I told him I hated taking my herbs and he told me how the Tibetan monks believe it's not the leaves that have been clipped, dried and ingested that have curative effects, but it's the relationship between the live plant and the patient that is beneficial. After he told me that, I decided to quit taking my herbs.

"In the morning, before you get out of bed, try licking your arm where it is painful," says David. "There are many curative agents in your own spit that may help that arm. That's why animals lick wounds when they get hurt."

"Lick it?" I ask. I think he just said, "Lick it."

"Yes, first thing in the morning before you get out of bed when your spittle is most concentrated," he tells me.

"Alright, I'll lick it, but that advice is pretty nuts," I tell him.

That night over dinner, I tell Jack about my licking plan.

"Well, it's worth a shot," he says. "It's more advice than your oncologist gave you. Why not?"

"Yeah, why not?" I drift off. "I'll lick it."

What the hell. It can't hurt, I think and I lick my arm with the funked-up vein the next morning.

I shit you not, in three days, the pain, the swelling, the redness, even the funky little BBs ... disappear. Score WooWooVille!

CHAPTER 17

Checkmate

As I understand it, our stem cells create our blood, which is comprised of white blood cells, red blood cells, leukocytes, platelets, gin and chocolate chips. A normal drop of blood has 3,500 to 10,500 white blood cells. But when you're in Candyland, things can get a little wonky and your stem cells can get bedraggled with all the nuclear bullying and toxic force-feeding. And then those stem cells go on strike and refuse to put everything into the recipe.

Apparently, we have pushed this game far enough and my stem cells are on strike, refusing to produce white blood cells and leaving me with about 1,000 white blood cells in a single drop of blood — 2,500 cells shy of what my blood needs to be considered healthy.

Is this going to kill me? No. But it does mean that I can't have my second round of chemo until my blood evens out, which could be weeks or months. It also means that during this time, I am in moderate danger of developing infections as my blood takes off its boxing gloves and hits the bench to catch its breath.

This isn't surprising, and I know it's a constant challenge in Candyland. Still, I'm so focused on finishing treatment and returning to life that this is just an irritating delay. It would be less irritating if it meant I could have a hall pass for a few days to normal life, but I'm sure my doctor won't approve that. I really want to join Jack on his upcoming trip to Texas where he will inspect his latest smoker (this one the size of a small train caboose), catch up with his buddies in the meat sciences department at Texas A&M, where he went to college in the '80s, and where he also went to Barbecue Summer Camp last summer, and hit some of his favorite barbecue joints. At my next appointment, I rhetorically ask my oncologist if I can fly.

"Sure, you can fly," he says. "The bacteria that pose a danger to you now are the bacteria in your own body, not external ones."

"Seriously?" I ask. "I've always heard when your blood count is low you shouldn't fly."

"You should be fine," he reiterates. "In fact, a vacation would probably be good for you."

This temporary stay from chemo with the doctor's blessing ignites my desire to buck up and get out of Dodge. Stepping outside of Candyland and witnessing growth and change for the future is not only fun, it's as if it establishes that there is a future. And besides, I love watching Jack chase his dream. Though he's still paying the family bills by working as a consultant in high tech, he's so ready to unlock his golden handcuffs, step to the edge of a cliff, and fly. He is exhausted by my Candy, working a job, tending to all of Rosemary's parenting, and trying to open his own restaurant. He needs a vacation desperately.

"Want me to go to Texas with you?" I ask him.

"Hell yeah!" he says, his Southern drawl thickening. "I would love to have you along. If you're serious, pack your bags baby. Let's giddy-up on down to Texas!"

It's been four months since I've ventured beyond appointments and cabin fever has set in. The thought of sunshine, Tex Mex and margaritas in the middle of December sounds like the perfect antidote to rain, chard and green tea.

"Let's do it! I'll go with you! Rose can watch the dogs and we can have a mini-vacation!"

When we get home, our gazelle is sitting in the living room drinking tea and reading a book.

"Rosie?"

Rose looks up from her book.

"If I go to Texas with Dad, can you watch the dogs?" I ask.

And miracle of all miracles, she lights up.

"Sure," she responds. "You should take a break."

Hmmm. Well that was easy, I think.

"You won't have any big parties or anything?" I ask. I don't know why I ask that. She's never been 'the partying type.' But leaving a high school senior alone for a long weekend touches my very tenuous responsible-mother bone.

"No?" she says, wrinkling her nose as if I just pooped on the floor.

"Sorry, I just have to ask," I say, feeling a twinge of guilt for the mere suggestion that she might be irresponsible.

"Are you sure you don't mind?" I ask.

"I'm sure. Go. I'll be fine."

God, I love that girl. She's so level-headed.

Days later, we fly over the Cascade Mountains, the Rockies, the Midwestern flatlands and arrive in the rolling hills that comprise the Texas Hill Country. Exhausted but exhilarated, I step out of the airport and drink in the warm dry air.

Jack's childhood friend David Berry picks us up from the airport and drives us to his home in Conroe, Texas. Hailing from a family of 11 children who grew up in White Rock Lake in Dallas behind Jack's childhood home, David and Jack share many memories since they played together as children.

I'd only met David a few times over the past 25 years, but hanging out with him is a true cultural experience. He is a rolling monologue of Texas one-liners.

"Tamina is a Texas town that should be in Arkansas," he tells us as we drive around our first morning looking for a breakfast spot. "He who dies with the most cars in his yard wins."

As we pass a potential breakfast joint, Jack asks, "Compadres, is that open for breakfast?"

"Yeah it's open, but he wants $4 for two eggs," says David. "At that price, I'll just steal them out of my neighbor's chicken coop."

We keep driving over railroad tracks and past strip shopping malls. We end up at Taquerias Arandes, where they have a dish called "Huevos Divorciados."

"It's two eggs separated by frijoles and steak because they're getting a divorce!" David laughs. "Jack, you know up in Fayetteville, they say, 'Hey, if I divorce you, are you still my sister?'"

As we drive back to his place after breakfast, David plans out our day. "After my son's football game, I'll let you taste my deer sausage with our steaks tonight," he promises. "You are going to shit a brick."

I spare him the details of my brick-shitting experiences of late.

Our friends Kat and Mike have flown down from Seattle to join us on this leg of the trip.

Our tour carries us to Texas A&M next. Jack is like a proud daddy with his new 13,500-pound steel offset smoker. We all jump in David's one-ton diesel truck and drag Leroi, Jack's name for the smoker, to College Station Texas.

"It's great that you're taking something so special from Texas to the Pacific Northwest," says A&M's Dr. Jeff Savell while 'christening' the smoker. "You have the passion — not just to feed yourself — but to feed people out there. It's like spreadin' the word of a missionary."

"Thank you, guys," Jack effuses. "Barbecue Summer Camp changed my life, literally. I can't thank you enough. It's so fun that I'll be feeding the people of Seattle. They'll come to know the work of the Texas barbecue."

I'm beginning to feel like I'm at a revival. *This would never happen in Seattle*, I think.

"On behalf of Texas A&M University and the barbecue geniuses here — Ray Reilly and Davey Griffin and me and all the students and grad students — we wish you nothing but the best, and we hope every brisket turns out and that you'll always have wonderful weather and it never rains on you."

Jack's BBQ a success? I'm a believer.

Never raining on him? Not gonna hold my breath.

Nobody asks about my bald head hiding under hats. Nobody looks at me with sympathetic pity. Nobody knows my secret. And it is SO nice!

We wrap up our trip touring around central Texas with Kat and Mike in a swirl of 100-year-old barbecue pits belching out the juiciest briskets, sausages and ribs that the world offers. For the first time in four months, I drop my teetotalling with abandon and have a margarita … or two.

When we return in Seattle (dogs still alive and no evidence of parties), Kathy is pulling me.

I cop a ride to Kathy's with my cousin Ada, who has moved to Seattle from Albuquerque to help me maneuver my brave new world.

Entering the foyer, Janice stands and hugs me.

"Deirdre! How are you?" she asks.

It's been more than three weeks since I've been here and I feel no small guilt over my absence.

"I'm fine," I tell her. "How's Kathy?"

"She's doing well, but her hip is still hurting her," she fills me in. "You know she's using a walker now so she's more sound on her feet."

My mother, graduating from a cane to a walker, seems so old-lady pathetic.

"Where is she?" I ask, looking around.

"In the living room. There's a singalong going on now."

"Oooh, I love the singalongs!" I tell her, sublimating my sadness that Kathy is becoming decreasingly ambulatory.

Ada and I head into the living room where Kathy is sound asleep in her chair. A walker sits next to her.

"Mom," I whisper into her ear. "Mom. Wake up!"

"What," she opens her eyes as if I just clocked her over the head. "Fart and be damned! What's going on?"

"Mom, Ada and I are here," I say.

"Oh, it's so good to see you two turds," she says as I give her a bear hug. "Who are you?"

"I'm your daughter, D-D, and Ada is your niece," I smile at her.

"Shit, I know that," she fakes. "Where the hell have you been?"

"I went to Texas, it's a state in the southern U.S.," I say.

"I know where Texas is, that's where I was born," she says, setting me straight.

Actually, my mom's from Utah. Details details.

"Hey, listen," I say, pointing to the singer in the middle of the room who's belting out "Chattanooga Choo Choo" with a karaoke setup. "You know this song."

"I do," she says. And she does.

"Pardon me boys, but that's the Chattanooga Choo Choo," she belts out without any prompting.

"Track 29," I join in. "Boy you give me a line!"

We muddle through a couple of songs, joining in the choruses and letting the karaoke guest sing the majority of the lyrics. When he finishes, I turn to Kathy.

"That was fun, huh?" I ask.

"Eh, it was alright," she states flatly.

"Hey, I made reservations at a restaurant," I fib. "Wanna go to lunch?"

"Hell yes," she says, "I'm hungry as a bear."

As I help her stand, placing her hands on her walker, we walk side-by-side to the dining room. Ada joins us and we sup on tomato soup and crackers.

"What's this?" asks Kathy, pointing to my purse.

"It's my purse," I tell her.

"Is this where you keep your marijuana cigarettes?" she asks.

One of my mom's little secrets while I was growing up was that she loved weed.

"Boy, I'm stuffed," I say, shifting the conversation and helping her stand when lunch is over. "Shall we go home and take a nap?"

"Yeah, I guess," she says. As we 'go home' (upstairs to her room), Kathy stops and looks at me.

"Where's Fred?"

"Who's Fred?" I ask, curious to know where her husband resides in her memory now.

"He's my uncle," she tells me. "He fought in the war."

"Oh, Uncle Fred," I answer. "Unfortunately, time caught up with him and he passed away a year ago."

"Is that so? Nobody told me," she says. "He was a good man."

"Yes, he was," I concur.

"Just up and died in his sleep one night," I tell her.

When we reach her room, I gently settle Kathy into her bed, draping the covers over her shoulders.

"I'm going to the potty and then I'll come join you for a nap," I tell her.

"Oh good," she says. "Who are you?"

"I'm your daughter, D-D," I tell her.

"I knew I liked you," she says.

"I'll be right back to snuggle. Close your eyes and go to sleep."

"OK kiddo," she says, relaxing into her pillow. "Hey kid, bring Arthur here."

"I will Mom," I say. "I'll be right back — with Arthur."

I leave her apartment and find Ada.

"OK Ada," I choke, "let's go."

Another life marker is unfolding in the Timmons' household. Today, Rose is taking her driver's test.

Jack stresses Rose out when he helps her drive, so she's requested a third party to step in. Michael, a friend of mine who's known Rose since she was 6, has been with her all morning, running through parallel-parking and backing-around-a-corner drills.

Like witnessing Jack starting a restaurant, watching Rose maneuver her latest challenge makes me feel that all the world has not just stopped and become one big sick fest. Rose will some day go to college. Maybe she'll get married and buy a house. Hopefully, she'll have a child or two. And though this is just a driver's license, it inspires a whole series of life projections in my mind that Rose will face and conquer, whether or not I'm around.

I vow to myself that if I do pass on, I will become Rose's guardian angel. I simply will not leave her. Though I've quit asking everyone I know about their spiritual beliefs, I have created my own novice belief system that the end is just a transition to some great unfathomable beyond where I will be able to shadow my loved ones until they no longer need me, at which point I will be released to the Universe and all of its wisdom in an infinite ascension.

Sounds pretty good, doesn't it?

Driving tests are taken at driving schools in Seattle now. You make your appointments in advance and everybody's kind and supportive at the testing centers. I don't know, without the obdurate DMV official judging your paltry youthful driving, it just seems too nice and easy.

"In my day ...." I want to tell Rose. But I figure at this time she doesn't want a history lesson on how much we suffered under the judgment of stern DMV officers who would fail you for the teeniest infraction. She is nervous, to say the least. Michael and I hug her as she heads out the door with her tester. I can feel the tension in her body.

Twenty minutes later she returns. With an ear-to-ear grin stretching her cheeks, Rose waves a piece of paper — the results of her test.

She passed. My baby is now a legally bona fide Washington state driver.

Check.

We text Jack a photo of Rose holding her temporary license. He texts us back the news that he has garnered his final investor and he can buy the restaurant.

Check. Mate.

CHAPTER 18

The immaculate conception

I haven't had my period in months. Hot flashes, followed by cold flashes, have become a regular, most irritating symptom. Hat, coat, scarf, sweater come off for three or four minutes at least five times an hour. Sleep has become elusive, as I wake throughout the night drenched in a pool of sweat. I throw off the covers and gasp for air, sometimes dripping water from my bedside glass onto my stomach, face, neck and arms to cool down. Then an arctic blast hits me as the ensuing cold flash plunges me into a seeming bucket of ice and I draw the covers back over my shoulders and sidle up to Jack's warmth.

As I gain weight from the steroids, my figure is changing. But I'm not just getting heavier — I'm aging in fast motion. My waist is thickening. The skin on my arms, legs and stomach is getting crepe-y and dimpled. Fine lines score my face with mind-numbing speed.

And then, there's sex — or lack thereof. Feeling like an ice pick is being rammed up me lady bits, the mere act of midnight coitus has become insurmountable.

"Ah, get out," I cry in pain when Jack tries to enter me. "Ow! Ow ow ow ow!"

Jack is generally patient with this new coital abstinence, but I know he will hit a wall. I feel ashamed that I can't offer him conjugal affection and I wonder how long this will last — or how long he will last.

I want to say, "It's OK, honey. Just have an affair while I'm like this." But I know that would break my heart and it would eventually destroy a marriage we've been building for 25 years.

"Is this permanent?" he asks in a genuinely curious tone.

"Shit I don't know," I say apologetically. "I'll ask the doctor what we should do."

After a few weeks' vacation from chemo, my white blood cell count is strong enough for my second round of chemo.

"How are you doing?" asks my oncologist before sending me up to the chemo ward.

"I can't have sex," I blurt out. Jack is in the room and remains silent, probably embarrassed by this frank announcement. "And my hot flashes are unbearable."

"It's not uncommon for chemo and radiation to incite early menopause," he tells me. "Are you having your period?"

"No, I haven't had it in months," I tell him. "Is … is this permanent? I mean, I'm in a marriage. I would like to have sex again."

"It's too soon to tell," he says. "Some women start menstruating after treatment, but at your age, you may not."

"And the hot flashes and the painful sex?" I press on. I feel like he's skirting the issue.

"That's not my territory," he admits. "This would be a good time to meet with your gynecologist."

My gynecologist, I think. *I haven't been to a gynecologist since Rose was born. I don't have a gynecologist.*

"I don't have a gynecologist," I tell him, taking off my coat as my temperature feels like it's reached boiling. "Can you refer me to one?"

"My nurse can get a name for you," he tells me.

I look at Jack, who's staring at a wall.

"Great," I say in a dull voice. "I'd like to be a little proactive."

"Look at the good news," the doctor tells me. "The protocol seems to be working."

True. I'm no longer dizzy as a bat, but I am dizzy as Lucille Ball — forgetting what I said to whom and when I said I'd do whatever it is I told people I'd do.

I learn they call this "chemo brain." It amounts to mental confusion and memory loss that can take years to shake and in many cases is permanent. Doctors don't know what causes chemo brain and quite conveniently, they don't know how to stop it.

"You will have no short-term memory after treatment," my radiation oncologist had told me during one of my early appointments.

"None?" I asked her.

"None."

"Ever?" I pressed on.

"Ever," she confirmed.

I was sort of bummed by that news, and by "sort of," I mean "very." I'm not the sharpest knife in the drawer, I'll be the first to admit. But I've always been at least smart enough to have a little career and raise a child (without doing too much damage) and achieve a satisfactory level of happiness. Having no short-term memory at 47 smacks too much of early Alzheimer's for my comfort. Yes, I want to return to health, but almost more importantly, I want to return to a baseline of intellectual fortitude that will allow me to remember my name and enable me to drive to the grocery store for milk and eggs.

Will I think Jack is my uncle some day? Will I remember that Rose is my daughter? Will I be Kathy's roommate at the memory home when this is all over?

Talking to a friend of Abby's, Jim, who survived Hodgkin's lymphoma against all odds, I ask him if the stupids that come from chemo fade with time.

"Not really," he tells me, "but it turns out you don't have to be that smart anyway."

Now, this is a gentleman who received a perfect score on his SATs and who's now midway through his Ph.D. in computer science, so he clearly had some IQ points to squander. "He's still completely capable and very smart," notes Jim, his good friend. "But he's softer and easier to be around. Cancer took the edge off — sometimes a knife can be too sharp."

But it made me ponder the intellectual afterlife following treatment.

If the chemo fog doesn't completely lift when I'm finished, what will I be capable of doing? As it is, I've given up on learning anything technical. I swear, if I ask Rose one more time how to turn off apps on my iPhone she's going to snap. More often than not, I don't recognize people I've met in the past few years or I forget major events in the news or in my life. Worst of all, I miss the punchline of every joke.

I've never been any good at telling jokes. In fact, I've always been REALLY good at ruining jokes. I mangle the setup. I forget the punchline, or I tell it too soon. My most common offense: I laugh so hard when it comes to the punchline, I can't spit it out. Then when I finally do — it's not nearly as funny as I've led my audience to believe it's going to be, and they're just disappointed by why the chicken crossed the road.

And to make matters worse, I love to tell — and ruin — jokes.

Then to make matters even worser, this Brain Candy fog means I often don't understand said jokes.

"Ha-ha-ha," people smile at me, patting me on the shoulder and exchanging subtle glances as they realize how off-track I'm running. "That's funny Deirdre. Good for you ..."

So when I received a card in the mail the other day, I don't think my friend could have anticipated what fire she was fanning when she included a couple of jokes in the card.

Me (reading the card): "What did the egg say to the pot of boiling water?"

Rose: "I don't know."

Me: "I can't get hard. I just got laid by a chick."

Then we both laugh. I nailed the setup. I didn't mangle or forget or over-laugh at the punchline. I told a joke with the finesse of Ellen Degeneres.

But wait, Chicken Lady. Don't count your eggs before they hatch! Because I can't leave a successful joke well enough alone, I add ...

"Though, I don't know why an egg would be talking to a pot of boiling water."

Then, Rose and I burst out laughing again. I got the delivery right. I got the punchline. I just didn't get the whole joke.

As much as I fear a future where I can't add two plus two or read anything longer than a photo caption, I absolutely dread a life without laughter. Even Kathy still has that.

Looking at the card, I catch my reflection in the mirror on our mantel.

"Rosie," I say.

"Yeah?"

"Come here," I say, still staring at my reflection..

"Why?" she asks.

"Just come here!" I tell her. "I want to show you something."

She heaves off the blue IKEA sectional and shuffles up to me. "What?"

"Notice anything?" I coyly ask, eyes bulging and suppressing a big smile. "Can you see it???"

"What?" she asks.

"Look at my head," I nod. "See it?"

"See what?" she again asks.

"Here, give me your hand," I say, taking her hand and rubbing it over my bald scalp. "Feel it?"

"Feel what?" she asks, completely befuddled.

"HAIR! I'm growing hair again!" I exclaim. "That's stubble you're feeling. Growing stubble!"

"That's great Mom," she says, a little underwhelmed for my taste.

"You bet your sweet ass it's great!" I stare in the mirror. "My doctor told me it would NEVER grow back and now it's starting to grow back. I'm gonna have hair again!!! Hello! Goodbye, featherless Chicken Lady!"

"Oh, weird," she says, now really inspecting my NEW hair. "Your skin is turning dark gray on top of your head."

"What?" I ask frantically. "What do you mean "dark gray"?

I grab a hand mirror and look at the top of my head. And wouldn't you know, just to ruin the moment of getting hair, I find out my scalp is countering the new hair with a sickening symptom — dark gray (dying?) skin.

"Actually, I think your eyebrows are doing it too," Rose says upon deeper inspection.

I shove my face to the smaller mirror and sure enough, the skin under my former eyebrows, which fell out weeks ago, is turning dark gray too.

"Google, Google," I gasp. "I need the Google. What new horror is this?"

I run to my computer and type in "dark gray scalp chemo." It pulls up a bunch of websites about how people's hair grew back in after chemo but it was a different color or a different type of hair, but nothing on the scalp actually going necrotic. I frantically call one of my nurses and leave a message.

"Hi, it's Deirdre. How are you?" I ask into the machine. "So, I just discovered the creepiest thing. My hair is coming back, yay, but my scalp and eyebrows are turning some kind of dark gray. Please can you tell me … what is that and should I be concerned?"

It's the first time during this whole trial that I've actually called a nurse on the phone for advice. I hang up and just look at my phone, willing it to ring.

It's not ringing.

Keep yourself busy, I tell myself, fearing that my head is now rotting and imagining not just a life with no hair, but a life with no scalp. I put some water on the stove to boil. I look at my phone. Maybe the ringer's off, I think. I check the phone — ringer's on. I return to the stove and open a package of Top Ramen. Then I stand in the kitchen willing the phone to ring and the pot to boil.

A watched pot never boils, I remember. So I leave the kitchen and my phone and I sit down in front of the TV with Rose.

"What are you making?" she asks.

"Top Ramen," I tell her. "It won't boil."

Rose, picking up on the fact that I'm acting a little more whacka-doodle than usual, goes into the kitchen.

"It's boiling," she informs me. "Want me to stir the noodles in?"

"Is my phone ringing?" I ask, which is a pretty thick question to ask since I would hear it ringing if it were ringing.

"Don't think so," Rose says. "Everything OK?"

And then, the phone rings.

I push myself up off the dining room chair and shuffle over to my phone. Glory be, it's the hospital calling!

"Hello, this is Deirdre," I blurt.

"Deirdre, hi, this is the nurse at UW," says a friendly voice. "I just got your message."

"My scalp is turning black! Do I need to come in? I can come in now. My daughter can drive me," I say, a little too fast.

"No, no, you're fine. That miscolored skin is where your new hair is pushing up from underneath the skin," she explains. "Congratulations."

Oh, but this is music to my ears. Glory hallelujah!

"Congratulations," I repeat, sinking into a chair. "He's a healthy bouncing baby boy."

My celebration is short-lived, as the game of "What Symptoms Persist/Worsen This Week?" continues. Numbness spreads from my hands and feet to my legs and back. Fatigue continues to make me look like a lazy sloth who will never get off the couch. Difficulty walking, getting out of cars, going down stairs, taking escalators (those are scary!), flipping from my back to my stomach in bed, getting out of bed, sitting on a toilet (without crashing into it), standing (yes, just plain old standing still), picking something up off the floor, opening cans, opening potato chip bags, texting, basically anything that involves using my hands or moving — becomes increasingly challenging. And this menopause business is turning me into a deranged woman, dressing and undressing throughout the day and night to accommodate my body's broken thermostat.

I try to find solace in the upcoming holidays. Since I can hardly stand without tipping over, Rose and Jack assume full responsibility for setting up and decorating the Christmas tree. Saul, the young British man who lived with us when I was diagnosed, has returned for the holidays and is now dating Rose. I take certain delight in showing off our country to him and his brothers, who are also visiting for the holidays, so we take them on our annual ski trip to Leavenworth, a charmingly cheesy faux Bavarian village in the Cascade Mountains. There's no snow this year, so we cook, they drink, and we all hang out in the hot tub in between televised football games. In an act of desperate boredom, we travel to a nearby town to bowl. I love to bowl. I don't do it often, but when I do, I'm kind of a master of the lane. Not to brag or anything, but, you know. Think again of Mary Catherine Gallagher on SNL and that's me. *Superstar!*

I pull on my striped leather shoes and start looking for 'my ball.' As I pull out a sparkly purple one, it weighs a ton. Move on. There's a ruby red one; it calls to me. Christ, I think, this one weighs a ton too. There's a hot pink one in the corner, probably a woman's ball at an appropriate weight for the daintier sex. It's perfect, except the finger holes are the size of a straw.

"That's a child's ball," says one of the workers dropping off our beers.

"Oh, I know," I lie. "We have a child joining us momentarily."

"You're up," Rose tells me. I'm gonna show Saul and his brothers how this bowling thing is done in America. *Superstar!*

I swagger to a (not pink) three-ton ball, wink at Rose, line up, slide forward, and drop/roll/throw my ball right into the gutter.

"I haven't played in forever," I say, explaining that perplexing throw.

My right side simply is not cooperating. I toss my second, third, tenth, twelfth throw exactly the same way, down the left gutter every single time for a total score of zero.

I try to laugh off my epic failure.

"Haha. So funny. Zero score," I snicker out loud. "Really, so funny."

I can't even roll a ball? What the fuck?

On the drive back to our cabin, I mask my embarrassment. "Look at that beautiful river," I say to the posse. "Gorgeous, huh?" *I mean, bowling? That's the easiest sport on Earth. I know how to bowl. Why couldn't I bowl? God dammit,* I think. *When I get home I'm going to bowl every fucking week till I can knock out at least one pin. Fuck fuck fuckity fucking tumor!*

I vow not to let the visitor in my brain get to me. I can beat something that's the size of a plum. *Watch me, Sara! You can't scare me. I've blasted you with radiation and poison — you're gonna lose this battle. The jig is up. Pack your bags and catch the next train out of Dodge ... and leave my balance at the door!*

I'll show her. I decide to rest up and tackle a skiing trip at our friends' Monica and Dick's upcoming wedding in Sun Valley. The plane ride is easy enough. There's a hefty line at airport security, but beyond that, I just have to sit on a plane. And if I'm strong enough to grow hair and fly, I'm strong enough to ski.

Screw bowling. It's a stupid sport anyway.

I'm going to hit the trail in Sun Valley and defy the cancer gods' grip on my coordination and I'm going to crosscountry ski. That's right, c-r-o-s-s-c-o-u-n-t-r-y-s-k-i. I can do this. This I can do. I've been skiing all my life and shooshing on cross-country skis is like crawling. Even toddlers can do it. I'll show those fancy Sun Valley social climbers what a true cancer-fighting warrior can do.

After settling into our cush digs, I take Jack's arm and together we stroll to the ski rental office.

"Five feet eleven inches," I tell the rental clerk for my cross country skis.

"And your weight?" she asks.

Though I've gained at least 10 pounds since my super-skinny just-call-me-Kate-Moss cancer low, I'm still much thinner than my usual self, and I still don't want Jack to hear what I weigh. I never have. It's none of his business and my weight has been a source of shame my whole life (thanks, Kathy). "Schpewe-schpewe-schpewe," I whisper into her ear. "Don't write it down," I tack on. I'm pretty sure Jack will have to sign off on our paperwork.

Jack grabs our skis and poles as I hold on to him for balance. We walk to the beginning of the nordic trail, which is right in front of an outdoor café where stylish families sip hot cocoa in front of an outdoor fire.

"Can you help me?" I ask Jack, whom I introduced to skiing twenty-some years ago.

"Yeah," he says, bending over my skis and locking my left foot in, and then my right foot.

"Wait," I tell him. "I have to hang on to you for balance. Hand me the poles."

He does and when I have both poles stretched out to my sides for balance, he puts his own skis on, wrapping his gloved hands around his poles.

"Ready?" he asks.

I look at the stylish crowd dining outside. It's not crowded on the trail. In fact, we're the only skiers out right now because apparently everyone is having lunch in that café. They look like extras in a James Bond film somewhere in the Swiss Alps. I'm kind of pumped to show off my mad sking skills in front of them. *They're probably just posers*, I think to myself.

"Ready!" I tell him.

He shushes forward. I side-step into his ski tracks and fall over. I can't get up.

"Jack!" I yell. "I can't get up."

He turns around and slides back to me asking, "What happened?"

"I don't know. I think my ski caught on the track or something," I wonder. "Can you help me up?"

Christ. How humiliating. All fashionable eyes are on me.

"Thanks," I say, avoiding looking at the café. "OK, let's go."

Jack turns around and starts flying down the path again. I slide my right foot out and fall down.

"Jack!" I yell again. "Help!"

He comes back. He lifts me up. I slide my left foot forward this time — and immediately fall.

I cannot ski. Something is so disconnected in my brain and body that I cannot accomplish the simple task of sliding one foot forward and then sliding the other foot forward.

Horrified, frustrated and madder than I've been since this whole fucked-up 'adventure' began, I burst out crying, throw my poles down, unsnap my bindings, and try to stand — only to struggle like an upside-down cockroach.

I am no longer OK with this whole cancer-taking-a-break-from-life-upbeat-YAY journey. I. Am. Pissed.

"Well, help me up!" I yell at Jack.

"Honey …" he starts to say while helping me up.

"Don't 'honey' me!" I scream. "This is FUCKED! Go ski by yourself!"

I try to stomp through the snow back to the resort. I weave and wobble, almost falling several times. I look at the café society, who are watching the scene.

Fuck you beautiful people! I think. *Just … fuck you!*

◎ ◎ ◎

Back on the waterlogged terra firma of Seattle, I vow to take this ride into my own hands. Again.

I go off all my medications and indulge in as many martinis as I feel I deserve. *Maybe the gin will kill Sara,* I muse, *because healthy things like bowling and skiing certainly aren't helping. Denial and self-destruction, please, come join me.*

I go off my Ambien and steroids and anti-nausea pills. What were they doing for me? Nothing, as far as I can see. Can't sleep. Can't bowl. Can't ski. Can't add two plus two. Can't skip, jump or run. Can't go up stairs. Can't stay warm. Can't stay cool. Can't menstruate. Can't shit. Can't even fucking have sex. At this rate, I will be my mother's roommate, and soon.

Screw the drugs. They're clearly not doing anything but damage. I'm sick of all this medicating for my medications. I'm done. Just give me the rest of my chemo and let's call it a day, folks.

I go drug free. I'm sure my doctors would say it's OK … if I consulted them. What do they know? They don't have to swallow all these dreadful pills and not take a shit for 14 days. But I do and I hate it and I'm not gonna do it anymore. Besides, everyone knows steroids make you fat and Ambien's addictive. I'm just gonna take a chance and go renegade!

"I've gone off my steroids again," I brag to my friend Alycia, who has a master's in nursing and fifteen years' experience as a nurse. "And in other news, feeling pretty bad overall."

"Did your doctor tell you to cut the steroids?" she asks.

"Well, no, not exactly," I kinda sorta tell the truth.

"OK, Deirdre," she says, staring me straight in the eye, "Swelling in the brain can cause permanent brain damage, and steroids keep that swelling down. You really need to either go back on them or tell your doctors what you're up to."

Alycia can be such a killjoy. Play by the rules. Do what your doctors tell you. Sit. Stay. Roll over. Alycia — teacher's-pet Alycia. My-shit-don't-stink Alycia. What does she know? Master's in nursing. So what? I have a master's in CANCER!

But I'll tell you something: The notion of permanent brain damage is enough to get me back on the wagon (or would that be "off the wagon" if you go back on drugs?) and start 'using' again.

Plus, not using wasn't nearly as great as I thought it would be. Two weeks into my new self-appointed drug-free regimen, no Ambien means no sleep and I feel like I'm suffering from sleep deprivation practiced on Cold War spies. The dizziness staved off by the steroids has returned, and now a simple flight of stairs finds me grasping stair railings like life rafts on the Titanic. I'm confused by simple instructions like a child at his first day of school.

So, for the second time, I go back on my pill and herb regimen.

And I tell everyone, "If you ever hear me say I'm going off something again without consulting the people in white coats, slap me. Hard."

Just as I get my sleep and dizziness back in order, I notice my breasts are swollen and sore, for like, the second week in a row.

Then, I think how I haven't had my period in months (my doctor said this can happen during treatment).

Then, I think how often I'm nauseous (they said this can happen during treatment).

Then, I think how I am ALWAYS hungry and have gained weight during chemo and radiation (they said this can happen during treatment).

Then, I think how I am always tired (they said this can happen during treatment).

Then, I think how my belly is swollen and distended (constipation, gas, steroidal weight gain?).

Then, I think how I crave foods I have heretofore never loved (like processed carbs and anything sweet).

Then, I think how I crave strange foods and how I have a sudden and very suspicious distaste for alcohol.

Then, I think, *This isn't cancer ... I'M PREGNANT!*

The same symptoms occurred 17 years ago.

"God, my boobs hurt," I told my mom over lunch years ago. "Look how big they are!"

"Hmmm," was all she said.

"And tired. I am tired all the time!" I exclaimed. "And I quit drinking out of nowhere, but I'm still hungover every morning."

"When was your last period?" she asked.

"Jeez, I don't know. I never pay any attention to that," I tell her. "I mean, it's like a surprise every month."

"You're pregnant," she matter-of-factly stated.

"Ha! That would be funny. But I don't think so," I said, while secretly wondering when my last period was.

After our lunch date, I kissed my mom goodbye and swung by the pharmacy to buy a pregnancy test. Before sitting on the toilet, I looked in the mirror. I was 29. My career as a newspaper reporter was just taking off. It took me years to break into reporting and this certainly would be an inopportune time to interrupt my career. But we had been married for seven years and I wasn't getting any younger, so, why not? After all, I did want children some day. Why not today?

I took a deep breath and opened the box, removing the test. If a line appeared I would not be one person, I would be two people. 'I' would be 'we.'

Freaky, I thought.

I released my bladder and plunged the stick into my urine stream.

I pulled the stick out, thinking I'd have to wait three or four minutes for the result. In the short time it took to lift the stick to my eyes, the line was there. I was pregnant. As it turned out, I was four months pregnant.

Today, realizing many of my symptoms are exactly in line with those I experienced 17 years ago, my thoughts go into a tailspin.

Oh my God, what if I am pregnant? I couldn't finish treatment. And then what if I relapse right away because I couldn't finish treatment and I die all of a sudden, leaving Jack with a baby? Or what if I don't finish treatment and I don't relapse but I get Alzheimer's like my mom and I can't count from 10 backwards by the time my child graduates from high school? Or what if I don't relapse and I don't get Alzheimer's, but my baby is born with three legs and one eye on the back of its head because it developed in a nuclear bomb site while swigging chemo cocktails? Or what if I don't relapse and I don't get Alzheimer's and I don't birth a three-legged-eye-in-the-back-of-its-head love child, but I just don't like being a middle-aged mom?

Then, I get all weepy, because I've always wanted a second child, which Jack and I tried for but The Fates didn't grant us, and I'm just giddy at the thought that we could have a baby just as Rose is abandoning us for her own life. And in my head, I start decorating Rose's former nursery for her cute wito bwover or sishter, and I start thinking how much better of a mother I will be the second time around because now I am SO wise.

Then, I get even weepier thinking we could not let this happen because of all the 'what ifs' and everyone would advise me to have an abortion and that would be the wise thing to do but, dammit, I want to have my baby! I DON'T WANT AN ABORTION!

Then my cousin Ada arrives and, witnessing the insane mental looping I'm caught in, she puts her foot on the brakes, "Why don't you just take a pregnancy test to find out before all this speculation?"

Oh. Yeah. That seems so sensible.

We drive to the pharmacy, grab an EPT and rush back home. I race into the bathroom with my little paper bag and pull out my wand of fecundity. I'm gonna have a baby! I'm gonna have a baby! I quietly sing to myself.

Excited at this, this MIRACLE and where it will lead me, I place the plastic stick in my urine stream, pull it out, and wait with a shit-eating grin on my face.

Barely ten seconds pass when I learn the heart-breaking news: Not pregnant.

Burp.

Of course I am not with child. And really, thank God. I mean, I love squishy babies and gangly children and petulant teens, but that's in my past. Still, a little part of me was furiously excited at the notion of a chubby little Phoenix rising out of my crispy burnt radiation ashes. Bereft, I shed a few tears and console my barren womb with some of Ada's ruby red borscht and take a long nap.

I have a new favorite thing: Monday luncheon.

When energy and schedule allow, I head to Kathy's care home on Mercer Island for lunch with the ladies.

At these luncheons, we abandon reason, step through the Looking Glass, and hop on our own little fantasy train. We ignore pop culture and current world affairs — except for the weather. The weather is our touchstone of reality — proof that we are among the living. The rain, the sun, the snow, they indicate that we are sharing a collective experience. We are not alone.

Over split-pea soup, egg-salad sandwiches, vanilla ice cream and decaf coffee, we leave one foot wobbily planted on Earth, freely floating the other foot in a past of bent memories and a future where we won't exist.

And lucky me, I get to be the conductor of this surreal ride!

Maude and Priscilla and Lucinda and Mom are the regulars at our lunches in the upstairs 'bistro.' The round table — adorned with fake flowers and a polyester white tablecloth — is surrounded by a curved bank of windows overlooking Mercer Island, Lake Washington, Bellevue and the Cascade Mountains.

Maude has forgotten where she's from today. So I switch tracks to reanimate her history as a ballerina and a model in Paris.

"Depuis quand habitez vous aux Etats-Unis?" *How long have you lived in the U.S.?* I ask her. I've noticed speaking Maude's native tongue wakes up her past.

"Pendant plusiers années." *For many years*, she answers. "Je suis venus pour danser." *I came here to dance.*

My mother interrupts.

"D-D, what did they do about all this?" she asks, circling her index finger toward my head. She is asking about the missing hair under my hat.

"I have brain cancer, but they've cured it," I tell her. There's no use in discussing cure rates and remission and relapse and all that. It would make her sad, and the last thing I wanna do is bring down the party. "The medication made my hair fall out, but it's growing back."

"That man came onto the unit today and asked how you were," she remembers. *OK, so Kathy was at work today.* "I didn't know what to tell him."

"Oh, was that John?" I ask, making up a man and rolling with the fact that Mom's been at work as a nurse today.

"Yeah, I think so. He likes you," she answers.

"Definitely John then," I answer, conjuring up a 'John' in my head. I think I'll make him a swarthy billionaire hopelessly in love with me. "How was work today?"

"Busy. Lots of heart attacks," Kathy shares. "Hey, your sister came by today," she continues, turning to Mary on her right. "She hates your sweater."

"My sister hates my sweater?" asks Mary, clearly hurt.

"Yeah, she hates it. She wants you to take it off. She hates that color."

Mary looks down at her sweater, running her right hand over her chest.

"Okaaaaaay," steps in the conductor to reset the track. "Beautiful day today, isn't it ladies? Look, everybody, you can see the Cascades. And the sun came out!"

As memories float in and out, I sense unseen guests — former lovers, fathers, mothers, friends, children — circumnavigate the table, touching a shoulder here, kissing a cheek there.

The funhouse feel of our almost reality makes my lunch companions fragile. Frustration can mount when they can't remember where they're from or if they have children or a spouse or a career, or even a name. The art of conversation on this trackless train doesn't involve follow-up questions — you just let a monologue run its course, often ending in a corner of confusion.

"Beautiful weather today! Look, you can see the Cascades! And it's sunny!" the conductor bubbles, resetting the tracks once again.

As the conductor, I can't indulge my Tourette's-like teasing — it confuses my passengers and hurts their feelings. And I certainly can't correct them or tell them they're repeating themselves. Instead, I straighten my cap and liberally toot the horn of flattery: "Your hair is beautiful today." "I love your slippers. They look comfy!" "It always makes me happy to see you!!" Just seeing their eyes light up with the simplest of compliments makes me feel like Mother Teresa (in the guise of Sinead O'Connor).

I evade certain personal topics, mostly marriage or children. Many of them have been married, but they've lost their spouses and reminding them of that can open a tragic book where nobody can remember the endings. Or they have children who may or may not visit them, but either way they won't remember when they last saw family and that will sadden them.

If things go seriously awry and one of my lunch buddies starts looping in confusion and sadness, I've discovered a 100 percent fool-proof remedy to a spiraling party.

"Hey, does anyone know the Andrews Sisters?" I ask. And then, I just start to sing "Rum and Coca Cola." Each lady friend joins in. The staff assistant Aster brings our ice cream. I comment on the Cascade Mountains outside. And we have one more smile at the beautiful sun before naptime.

CHAPTER 19

The never-ending slog

It's March. This will be my third chemo infusion since radiation ended — the first one in September, the second one in December (delayed a few weeks because of bad blood), and now my third infusion, which has been delayed three months because my blood is severely flagging with scant white blood cells. It's clear my body's not receiving the treatments with much strength and the threat that I will not be able to finish all nine sessions is very real.

The curiosity with which I first entered Candyland has faded. I discontinue meal train because I am tired of putting out my friends. I'm tired of visitors and deny most requests from friends who want to drop by. This all has been going on for more than 10 months, and I'm no longer intrigued by what happens to our souls when we die — I could give a rat's ass now. I just want to get this game over with. Everything hurts and I have nothing to talk about but TV reruns. What began as a frightening and exciting tightrope balance between life and death has become a long slow slog. And now that I've had a three-month respite from the toxic bombing due to my flailing blood, I'm getting a glimpse of life post-treatment.

Nausea is slowly dissipating. I can make it through a busy day with only a few hours of couch time to rest. Some of my strength and coordination are returning. I made a family meal for the first time in almost a year. My primary dizziness has eased and I've started driving again, which means I'm more independent.

So it is with mixed feelings that I hear my white blood cell count is just high enough to go at it again. Having gone from Vincristine once a week for five weeks (during radiation) to a couple of infusions of Cysplatin followed by a dose of Lomustine in a pill, the doctor is switching me to a two-day infusion (2700 milligrams total) of Cytoxan to see if that chemo allows my blood to recuperate more quickly.

I think they keep switching the chemos because some chemos kill some things, some chemos kill other things, some are really hard on you, and some are not so hard on you. So the fart smellers at the chemo clinic mix it up to keep my body guessing as the potpourri of toxins that root out hiding cancer cells and/or give my body a break when one chemo pummels me too hard.

It's kinda like dueling thugs attacking you in a back alley: Hey, quit stabbing her, she's going to bleed to death. Punch her in the face for a while. Yeah, yeah, now kick her in the shins!

Cancer is getting old, and I'm becoming very tired of this marathon in Candyland. And I'm tired in general. Even my visits with Kathy aren't providing their usual pick-me-up. It's been almost a year since she first moved to Sunrise. The last time we went to Starbucks she didn't understand where we were and her mocha latte was "horrible!" She never asks where Arthur is anymore. In fact, the last time I took him to visit her, she didn't know what he was.

"He's a dog," I told her. "He's your dog."

"Oh," was all she said.

Same with my dad. She rarely mentions him these days, and when I tell her he's passed on, she nods her head with a blank expression.

I guess I should be glad that she seems to enjoy Sunrise, but witnessing her complete cognitive disappearance shatters my heart.

My cousin Ada and I spend many days cleaning my childhood home. We've cleared out closets and cupboards and taken many trips to the Goodwill. Nobody from my family will live in this house again. We are grown up. We own our own homes. Even our children are grown up. It's time for the mid-1970s faux Tudor home overlooking a forest at the end of a cul-de-sac on a bustling little island to welcome a new family. Yet-unborn little feet can toddle around the hardwoods. Different kitchen aromas can sweeten the air. The neighbors can celebrate the Fourth of July with a new mom or dad lighting fireworks safely on the quiet little street.

But we are finished here.

I've unloaded most of the drawers and broken clocks and unworn slippers. My friend Daniel has updated the ochre and fake brass lighting with new fixtures, he's replaced brown and gold shag carpets with wool-blend Berber carpets, and he's painted the interiors, masking the cigarette-stained walls.

As Ada brings me boxes to go through, I sit on the floor and sort through the objects of my life — long-lost diaries, files marked "Private: DO NOT TOUCH" that carry old Teen Beat magazines; the dolls whose hair I cut and whose faces I burned on the cooktop when I was 3; the hand mirror that my mother held in bed every Sunday as the morning sun revealed the stray facial hairs that needed to be plucked; the many sets of reading glasses that my father kept around the house as his eyes aged; the unopened, unused Band-Aids that are now yellow with time. And the mouthguard. The mouthguard Kathy constantly misplaced as her Alzheimer's progressed.

I go downstairs and grab the Tupperware that my mother stored her mouthguard in. I run back upstairs and fill it halfway with water — as my mother always did. I place the mouthguard in the Tupperware. And I place the Tupperware on the windowsill, where it belongs … at least until the house is no longer ours.

As I slowly bid adieu to my childhood home, Jack returns to the property where he wants to house the future Jack's BBQ. That's right. It's official. Jack is going to open his restaurant. With the commitment from his final investor, he can now close the deal on the dive bar.

Though Jack still consults with a high-tech company, he spends evenings and weekends on the new space. In a matter of weeks, his burly group of ax-wielding, drill-drilling, hammer-smashing friends tear apart Bogart's walls, ceilings and floors, demolishing the dive-y sports bar.

Gone are the '80s mirrors. Gone is the sports memorabilia. Gone are the hurkin' TVs from the windows and walls. Gone are the chain-link fences delineating one seating area from another.

Windows that had long been obscured by particleboard and TVs are now opened back up to the sun (and, er, rain). Secret doors covered by corrugated steel are revealed and either restored or removed. Past faulty construction projects are exposed and repaired. And the unsightly pull-tab machines are sent packing.

I grab an old vinyl chair from the building's previous incarnation and sit in awe as the dedicated demolition team rips, strips and pulls apart someone else's dream and begins to build a new dream.

Jack, our intrepid smoker, travels to Texas to collect smoking tips and industry tricks from pitmasters, butchers, farmers, ranchers — you name it — the Who's Who in Texas 'Cue. There's no backing out now. We have the keys, we are more than excited, and there are plans afoot that involve Seattle talent on many levels of food, drink, entertainment, and a good old-fashioned appreciation for down-home vittles.

By May, I'm buoyed by my many months of survival since that first diagnosis of certain death. I almost feel giddy about the prospect of finishing treatment and getting back to life as I know it. So, I take stock. How is the House of Deirdre?

I've gained a lot of my weight back, which pisses me off. No longer model-thin, I look like a regular Joe in the middle-aged mom figure department.

My hair and eyelashes and eyebrows are valiantly trying to grow back. Whereas I always had stringy sandy brown hair in the past, it's coming in soft and thick in a patchwork of curly gray and dark brown. After a lifelong habit of coloring my hair that my mother started when I was a child, I'm ready to wash that gray right out of my hair, so I visit my gal pals at Vidal Sassoon, and my colorist Abby gives me an auburn wash.

I look 10 years older than when this all started. That irks me.

Having been a Botox fan for years (I didn't mention that in my roster of "Why do you think you got cancer" question — but I have my suspicions), I'm ready to smooth out the furrowed grooves in my forehead that I inherited from my father.

Shut up. I know it's vain. Don't judge.

So I wrangle my friend Daniel to join me as I go to the cosmetic surgeon for my yearly forehead 'ironing.' As I fill out the exhaustive paperwork, on page 3 it asks, "Are you currently on any medication?"

Yes, I check.

"If so, list them."

Cisplatin, Lomustine and Cytoxan, I list.

On page four: "List any surgeries you've had and when you had them."

Brain biopsy, July 2013, I write.

"Are you currently undergoing any medical treatment?" it asks. "If so, for what?"

Yes, for brain cancer, I say.

Simple enough. I hand the paperwork to the receptionist and wait for them to call my name.

"Deirdre?!" calls a woman at the door, looking at me. Dan and I are the only two people in the lobby.

"'Tis I," I say, standing.

"This way please," she directs.

"Dan, come with me," I say, still not wanting to be alone during any appointments, even Botox.

"Hello," a friendly-looking gentleman says. "And you are …"

"Deirdre," I finish his sentence.

"And you're here today for …"

"Botox," I finish for him again, trying to be efficient with his time. "Forehead and between the eyes."

He takes a look at my forehead, eyeing it for where he'll place the needles.

"Have you had Botox before?" he asks.

"Many a time," I admit.

"OK, well, let's get started," he says, flipping through my paperwork.

He stops on page 3.

"Cisplatin, Lomustine and Cytoxan," he asks. "Is that a joke?" Then he flips to page 4. "You have brain cancer?"

"Well, hopefully 'had' brain cancer, but I'm still getting treated for it," I admit.

"What's your blood cell count?" he asks, incredulously.

"Hovering between one and two," I tell him.

"And you're here to get an elective invasive procedure?" He's starting to sound mad.

"Yes?" I say, bracing myself for a lecture.

"Get out of my office," he almost shouts, scribbling notes all over my paperwork.

"What are you writing?" I ask, now equally upset.

"I'm writing that you came into my office asking for an elective invasive procedure while under hard-core drugs and struggling with a serious life-threatening disease and that I'm kicking you out of my office!" He's now just yelling and scribbling HARD. "Get out!"

"Alright, I'll go I'll go," I say, sounding more than defensive. "Just … please stop writing!"

"Goodbye," he says.

"Wait, before I go," I press on, undaunted by his hysteria, "can you tell me what these are?" I ask, pointing to a series of weeping red spots that have been proliferating on my face.

"They're pre-cancerous lesions that need to be frozen off when you're HEALTHY," he says. "Now is not the time to deal with those."

"Will freezing them off scar?" I ask.

"Probably," he states, in a somewhat self-satisfied tone.

"Can you ..." I start to ask.

"No! Get. Out. Of. Here," he reiterates, still scratching notes in my file. "And don't come back. You shouldn't be doing ANYTHING like this until you are completely cancer-free with a blood cell count of at least 10. Botox with a blood-cell count of one! What are you thinking? Go!"

Dan and I stand up and leave.

"Hm, that went well," I say to Dan when we're safely in his car and driving home.

🍭 🍭 🍭

My steroids continue to inspire powerful cravings, most of which are for salty Asian dishes — oxtail *pho* filled with fresh basil and jalapenos, sushi drawn through a liberal bowl of soy sauce and wasabi, spicy Thai *pad see ew* with shrimp, *dim sum* dredged through pepper oil and soy sauce. All of this super-salty food then makes my mouth as dry as a popcorn fart, so I carry my Camelbak filled with water and sip from it constantly like a baby with a bottle.

Today, my brother Don and I are at one of my favorite Vietnamese diners, Moonlight. Sweeping the room with a glance, I see a party of six dressed in white robes, turbans and lots of gold.

I do a double take.

One of them catches me staring. I've never been very cool when I see something out of the ordinary (in this case, *someone* out of the ordinary) and I get kind of Touretty.

"What are you?" I ask.

"We're Sikhs," one of the women enthusiastically responds.

"Sikhs!" I say. "I've never met any Sikhs. What is ... all this?" I motion at their crazy cool apparel. They look like they've been pulled from central casting for a 1950s epic on the Holy Land.

"These are our garments," the lady tells me. "Have you never seen a Sikh?"

"Well, yes, but usually behind the wheel of a cab," I answer, immediately wishing I could rescind that statement.

"Perhaps," one of men laughs. "You should attend one of our yoga sessions to learn more about the Sikh culture in Seattle."

"Yeah, no, that's not gonna happen," I resolutely state.

"Why not?" one of the bearded gentlemen asks.

"Because I have brain cancer and I have no balance," I answer. I hate to admit it, but I've come to like sharing this very personal challenge. It's such a dramatic declaration and it carries such gravity, but when said nonchalantly, I think I come off as a sparkly bomb.

The man who had just spoken jumps up and pulls a chair next to me, putting his arm around my shoulders. It's kind of nice and comforting ... if a little forward.

"What are you doing for it?" he asks, almost touching his nose to mine.

"The usual, chemo and radiation," I tell him. "But I do other stuff too, Eastern stuff, like get massages and acupuncture and colonics."

Deirdre, why do you share the colonic thing? It's gross.

"May I offer you a very effective Ayurvedic treatment for brain cancer?" he asks.

He's so warm and he smells good. I wonder if that long beard smells good too, or if it smells like yesterday's lunch.

"Sure, tell me everything, *sensei*," I joke with him.

"Eat nothing but raw onions for six weeks and your tumor will die," he offers.

"Oh, yes. You see, I am not going to do that," I wholeheartedly confess.

"Why?" he asks.

"Nothing but raw onions for six weeks? That's why I'm not doing it. I HATE raw onions and besides, I'm sorry, that just sounds like a bunch of hooey," I tell him. "With all due respect."

"Ayurvedic medicine has been around for thousands of years. It was developed on the Indian continent and has a much longer history than Western medicine. Successful cancer treatments have been well-vetted," he instructs me, unfazed by my doubt. "But if you're unwilling to eat raw onions, then how about boiling onions and garlic and drinking the broth — and only the broth — for six weeks," he

271

says, as if this is a more palatable option. "But you can eat nothing else during this time."

"Strike two," I tell him. "Not goin' do it," I say in my best Dana-Carvey-cum-GeorgeBush accent.

"How about drinking your urine?" he asks. "Would you be willing to do that?"

"Oh, sure, that sounds fine," I joke. "Why didn't you just start with that treatment? I'll just go in the bathroom right now and handle up on a good frothy cup of my pee."

This guy's wack, I'm thinking. *What next? Back to the coffee colonics and vitamin C IVs that people pushed when I was newly diagnosed?*

"I know these suggestions sound unfamiliar, but these Ayurvedic treatments I'm recommending have been used to great success in treating cancer for literally thousands of years."

"Come on," I say. "If eating onions and drinking your pee cures cancer, don't you think everyone in the world would just do that?"

"Medicine is a high-dollar industry," he reasons. "You can't make money on onions and urine. What has your treatment cost so far?"

"I don't know," I tell him. "Hundreds of thousands of dollars?" I guesstimate.

"Right," he looks deeper into my eyes. "A lot of people are making a lot of money off you."

True dat.

"What are these?" he asks, pointing to my embarrassing facial lesions.

"Pre-cancerous lesions," I tell him. "I'm waiting for my white blood cell count to recuperate so I can have them burned or frozen off."

"At least do this," he continues. I'm working hard to secretly smell his beard. I don't think it smells like food. I think it smells good, like the rest of him. "Every morning during your first urine of the day, swab these lesions with your urine. It will cure those. And any other skin problems you have," he shares, looking at my prodigious acne breakout. "Your own urine is filled with anti-bacterial agents, enzymes, hormones, uric acid and minerals."

"OK, dude, I love the whole thing you got going on," I tell him. "Your clothes, your beard, your sweet smell. But your ideas are about the craziest thing I've encountered on this journey and I don't think I'll be bathing in — let alone DRINKING — my urine anytime soon. I don't care how 'proven over thousands of years' pee cocktails are. Sorry, you are barking up the wrong tree. Woof woof."

He gently laughs and gives me a hug before returning to his table.

"You can go online and read about it," he reasons. "Think about it. And when you feel ready, join our yoga group. We practice kundalini."

Isn't that the sex yoga? I think to myself. *Was that a come-on?* Looking back at the six robed people, I think, *That was like a journey to a mystical forest ... tripping on LSD.*

Drink my pee. As if.

The next morning as I relieve myself I think, *What the hell.* It can't hurt. I gag slightly and put a wad of toilet paper in my stream. I mean, it's totally yucking me out, but when I licked my weird chemo-damaged vein, it did work. Maybe, just maybe? While I can't envision drinking my pee, maybe I can try this wonky treatment of daily pee swipes across my lesions. I mean, it won't kill me. Right?

I swipe. I close my eyes trying not to wretch. I throw the wad into the toilet.

And here you go kids, I feel the lesions burning.

For the next three or four mornings, I do the pee swipe and wouldn't you just know … my lesions go away.

As my white blood cell count continues to flag, I'm denied chemo once again. I've only had three of my nine sessions over the past 11 months, and my doctor is now questioning how many more infusions I can tolerate. He decides to wait another month in hopes that my blood will at least hit the minimum numbers to support more toxicity.

Rose, who is halfway through her senior year in high school, faces college applications in a few short months. We have already visited schools in Europe after her junior year. With lower tuition prices outside of the U.S., we were hoping she'd fall in love with the Sorbonne or the University of London, even schools in Sweden or Taipei that we'd never seen but boasted super-affordable ticket prices coupled with great reputations. She vetoed our ideas, firmly stating that she wanted to attend college in the Midwest or the East Coast.

With nothing holding me here (except for my extreme fondness of the couch), Rose and I decide to travel to the Midwest to look at some of the colleges she's interested in. Having been born and raised in Kansas, it's been more than 30 years since I've been to the heartland and I'm curious to see how it's changed. Or if it has.

I grew up in a middle-class neighborhood in Wichita where the newest neighbor had only lived in their house for 20 years, while the rest of the residents had lived on the street since the '30s. The new-comers were referred to as "The Catholics" by the rest of the neigh-bors. On a street where everyone else was Methodist or Episcopalian, "The Catholics" were suspicious. Not only did they have (gasp) four children, but they always had the nicest driveway on the street. The weather in Wichita wreaks havoc on concrete, and keeping up with the cracks and concrete disintegration is costly. "The Catholics'" boastful display of a yearly repaving flaunted their financial security. Along with the divorced couple down the street who had inelegantly remarried and merged two families of children, "The Catholics" and "The Brady Bunch" were never invited to the neighbors' cookouts and cocktail parties.

Since both our parents were working, my brother Sam and I had a healthy list of weekly chores: trim the overgrown grass encroaching the driveway; unload and reload the dishwasher; vacuum the house; clean the bathrooms; dust the house; plus a rigorous dictate to prac-tice piano an hour a day. Sam and I would come home from school, poke at our chores, look at the piano, then descend to the basement where "Gilligan's Island" and "I Dream of Genie" offered a welcome escape from our boring chores, piano practice and homework. After frittering away hours watching TV, when we heard my mom's car pull into the (crumbling) driveway, we'd quickly turn off the TV and pull out our schoolbooks. That worked until my mother discovered she could feel the TV and if it was warm, she knew we'd broken the rules and skipped out on our obligations.

Food was a curious notion in our home. Well, this was the '70s in Kansas and I think it's pretty safe to say that food was a curious notion in most Midwestern homes. Ground sirloin, iceberg lettuce, American cheese and white bread were the norm. When Kraft Mac-aroni and Cheese came into our home, Sam and I nailed the recipe: Boil water, add noodles, drain noodles, open packet, pour cheese powder over noodles and add milk. That was our perfect meal. The more adventurous neighbors ate Rice-A-Roni, a Chinese dish in the guise of a San Francisco treat. We suspected "The Catholics" ate Rice-A-Roni — that would be just like them and their fancy ways.

Etiquette was paramount in Wichita, where "Please" and "Thank you" were burnished into our brains. At school, I had to wear dresses every day and Sam had to wear suits (it was a private school). Political correctness had no place in this land, where many businesses maintained back-alley "negro" entrances as a dark reminder of the past.

Rose and I aren't traveling to Wichita — we're going to Ohio. While I wonder how society has evolved in the heartland, I'm most excited to see if the mid-western diet has evolved since I left. Will there be pho and sushi and chai lattes? Or will we be faced with dry cheeseburgers and canned peas?

I'm not surprised to say, it is the latter. Our first meal at a diner serves us fish and chips, which should be called 'Filet O'Fish and soggy fries.' My 'diet platter' of Jello, chopped sirloin and cottage cheese should be dubbed "A Trip Down Memory Lane."

In Gambier, Ohio, we discover Hogwarts' U.S. subsidiary at Kenyon College. Built in 1824, the college's stone-and-stained-glass dining room is only surprising in that the chandeliers hang from the ceiling — instead of magically floating above students' heads. Truly one of the most beautiful campuses we've visited, the school opened its doors to female students in 1969. It hosts a Greek system with sororities and fraternities that cover a gamut of interests. Paul Newman and president Rutherford B. Hayes went here. Rose and I depart after several happily spent hours of walking the campus, meeting students, and dining in the elegant dining hall.

"Did you love it?" I ask her. I loved it.

"Meh," she says. "It's so white."

"You're white," I point out.

"Yeah, but it's whiiiiiiite white," she notes. Having grown up in a mixed Seattle neighborhood with a veritable potpourri of ethnicities, sexual orientations and economic variances, Rose is clearly discomfited by the lack of diversity.

As Hogwarts, USA, grows distant in our rear-view mirrors, we decide to take a break from tours and instead suss out some local history. With a quick click of The Google, we learn that we're only an hour away from an Amish settlement in Ohio's Coshocton area.

"Let's check out the Amish," I suggest. "We can take their pictures and steal their souls."

"Mom," she complains.

"I'm just kidding," I placate her. "But if you shoot them with your iPhone they probably wouldn't even know!"

"Seriously," she admonishes. "Stop it."

"God, you are no fun," I tease her.

As we approach a town called Roscoe Village, we pass an Amish man driving his buggy on the highway. I suppress the deep urge to ask Rose to pull out her iPhone and do some soul stealin'. Then we pass another Amish man snoozing in his parked buggy in a farm driveway. The sightings are kind of like spotting deer — only much more exciting. "There's one!" "Oh, quick quick quick, look over there. See the one sleeping in his buggy?"

"I wish we could see a female one," I say, as Rose sits in exasperated silence.

"When did you become the mom and I became the child?" I ask her, somewhat disappointed that she won't play Spot The Amish with me.

"When I was born," she says.

It's kind of true. Rose is a somber, responsible creature. She's the type of person who returns library books on time and is never late for anything. I, on the other hand, have struggled all my life with just remembering appointments, let alone being on time for them. My library card was revoked long ago for missing returns and unpaid fees. I'm most somber when sleeping — the rest of the time I'm cracking one-liners and quoting old vaudeville jokes.

I keep it to myself that I'm a little more than excited to see a whole herd of Amish in their natural habitat when we get to the village. Maybe we'll even get to see them in action, like, kneading dough or plowing the land or darning socks. When we check in at the small town's visitors' center, a woman in a long dress and a bonnet greets us, and I can barely contain myself.

She approaches Rose and me and asks if we have any questions.

Oddly, she has bleached her hair blond and she clearly wears makeup. I think to myself, *This one's a rebel!*

"Well, yes," I respond. "Please do tell me about your garments. They are Amish, I presume?"

I endeavor to sound old-timey for the lady. Instead of saying something like, "What are you wearing?" or, "Are those Amish clothes as uncomfortable as they look?" or, "Do you sew your own stuff by hand?" I speak in plain terms with no modern or crass slang.

"I'm not Amish!" she snaps back, acting as if perhaps I had deposited an accident on the hand-loomed rug. "This is Canal Era wear."

"Right!" I say, as if I'd just had a small stroke and she jogged my memory.

"From Erie Canal," she continues. "You know about Erie Canal."

"Oh yes! Erie Canal!" I answer, slightly embarrassed that I can't remember that elementary school lesson. "Um … what's Erie Canal?"

"The canal used to run under that freeway," she says, pointing to a nearby road and looking as if I had just crawled out from under a rock. "It cut across the length of Ohio in the 1800s, and horses attached to the boats on each side would pull them down the canal.

"Would you like to watch our video on the history of the canal?" asks the non-Amish woman.

"Of course! Yes! We'd love to see it!" I say.

Sheesh. She's so sensitive about this Canal business. I daren't say, "No."

So Rose and I follow the non-Amish sharp-tongued Canal woman into the Visitors' Center salon and she starts the documentary about the town's history. Written blow — by — blow, the film provides an exhaustive account about the town's founder who struck out with his bride after getting laid off in a nearby town and how they opened a glove factory and how .... OH! Wait, did I nod off or did you?

After what seems like 28 days have passed, Rose and I conspire to sneak out of the Visitors' Center, sheepishly peeking into the hallway and tiptoeing toward the door.

"How was it?" the woman emerges from out of nowhere.

We can clearly hear what must be the world's longest documentary still blaring in the other room.

"It was great!" I lie. "We can't wait to hit the Amish — I mean Erie Canal — town! Thank you!"

As her eyes narrow in acknowledgment of my lie, we head for the nearest exit.

"Bye! Thanks! Have a great day!" I belt out rushing through the door. "Bye!"

"If she'd been Amish, she would have been much sweeter," I tell Rose after we're safely away from the Center.

"Stop it," is all she says.

"Hey, I got us out of that pickle," I tell her.

"You also got us into that pickle," she counters.

As the mother of an only child, I feel that it is my parental duty to rib Rosemary from time to time. Since she has no siblings, I think it's only fair she learns how to handle playful teasing from me. I know. I know. You're probably thinking, "What conscientious mothering."

"Hey, let's skip down the street holding hands," I say, with a sudden burst of energy.

"No."

"Come on, Rose! What if I die and you think, 'Wow, all she asked me to do was skip down the street and I didn't do it,'" I tell her. "Then you'll be sorry."

"Mom, don't say that," she chides. "You know I hate when you say that."

"OK, then skip with me."

Reluctantly — very reluctantly — Rose takes my hand and we start to skip.

Correction: Rose starts to skip.

It turns out, that my coordination challenges extend to skipping, and the right side of my body can't jump up because of my tumor, Sara.

"Oh my God, Rose! Look! I can't skip," I say in amazement, flailing down the sidewalk. "Let me jump."

And it also turns out, I can't jump. My brain is simply not sending the signals that trigger jumping (and skipping).

"Whoa, weird," says Rose. "Are you doing that on purpose?"

"No, seriously, I can't do it," I say in surprised disappointment.

Suddenly, my playful mood shuts down. As I ponder how I can't bowl or ski or walk up stairs or go down an escalator or get out of the car without help or roll over in bed or skip or jump or anything. I feel deflated as I reckon with what I've become.

"Mom, it's OK," says Rose, picking up on my mood shift. "You'll get it all back."

"How do you know?" I ask her despairingly. "I'm like a 90-year-old woman."

"It's just temporary," she comforts me, taking my hand in hers. "It's OK."

I appreciate that she's intuiting my fear and reaching out to help me stabilize, physically and emotionally. She is doing what Kathy no longer can — she is comforting me in a very motherly way.

"Alright," I tell her. "Let's just hit some of the stores and head back."

So we hit the town. We buy homemade candy. We buy an old book. We take our picture in front of the curiously named North Whitewoman Street. After an hour or so I am completely tuckered out from our fruitless Amish watching. We beat it back to the sanitized-if-blasé comfort of electricity, clean sheets, sweat pants, microwave popcorn, Internet, and cable TV at our Hampton Inn suite in Elyria.

Since we are so close, the following day we take a sidetrip to Detroit to see the reputed haunting allure of rapidly rotting train stations, homes, factories, office buildings, theaters and streets. As we drive into the beat-up town, we are both immediately transfixed by the mixture of hope and despair. While columns crumble, windows break and walls fall, there is an undeniable rush of energy surging beneath the city's cracked and splitting soul. We hit Corktown, a tiny revolution of renovation with good restaurants and small shops — all under the shadow of the skeletal remains of the grand turn-of-the-century Michigan Central (train) Station. The Eastern Market is a colorful blast of energy with farmers and craftsmen, antiques dealers and artists hawking their products and wares. The Heidelberg Project pokes creepy fun at neighborhood decay, turning an entire residential block into a humorous nightmare of domestic memorabilia, clothing and outright trash adorning the decaying homes and yards. Pocket hotspots of craftsmen's shops, teahouses and yoga studios hide in renovated lofts, storefronts and basements. And while the city is screaming out for help as it tries to tread the dirty swamp of bankruptcy, the people are so kind, accommodating, warm and friendly that you would never surmise their city is teetering on the brink of financial and physical implosion.

I feel like the human embodiment of Detroit — broken down and falling apart. But that is only my body. My spirit has a deep undercurrent of hope and renewal, just like Detroit.

On our final day, we visit another charmingly tony college, Oberlin. We love the relaxed and friendly academic atmosphere and the comfortably diverse student body (it was the first college in America to integrate black students into the previously all-white college). There's a friendly air on campus and the one class we attend is intimate and lively with genuine student involvement.

"I could see going there," Rosemary shares on the plane home. "Kenyon was just too All-American jock-y for me, but Oberlin, yeah I liked it. But man, I don't know if I can handle the Midwest. It just seems so straight-laced. And the food ...."

Not wanting to study on the West Coast — probably because it's too close to us (?) — Rose and I plan one more college search trip in the fall to the East Coast.

We return from our trip in time for Rosemary and her buddies to prepare for the great American tradition known as prom.

Rosemary's 'date' is her childhood friend, Hadley. Rose and Hadley share a life-long history of performing home-made plays, whispering life secrets, negotiating academic challenges, taking family trips, and making short films together. While Hadley and Rose and a growing group of 17-somethings collect in our basement, the requests for glitter and hair pins float upstairs while I scrounge around for flat irons and hair pieces and pins and ribbons. Never having experienced prom (I attended a girls' school that did not partake in this celebrated rite of passage), I used to turn my nose up at the foreign teen passage known as prom. It just felt alien to me. But more than a year into the threat of missing major life markers, I am overjoyed to be alive and witnessing another of Rosemary's teenage rites of passage. Grabbing my best camera, I go to Rose's room to capture this little electric moment in life. In fact, think I'm more excited than the kids.

Eventually, other parents arrive, descending to Rose's already-crowded basement bedroom to relish in our progenies' varying stages of glamor and excitement. As we secret a little cash to our respective offspring and click photos of the epic preening, I sink into the unbridled joy of an interlude so simple as a high school dance.

CHAPTER 20

Nice ash

Amma is a spiritual leader from India who heads a worldwide faith and proclaims, "Love is my religion." Many of her devotees consider her a living goddess and believe a single hug from Amma's Motherly embrace can be healing and transformational.

Well, doncha know she's coming to Seattle?

"Do you want to see Amma?" asks Ada, who has received many hugs from Amma in the past.

"OK, if you insist." I tell her, secretly snickering at the folly of this whole hugging business. I'll let Amma hug the cancer out of me.

Several weeks later, we jump in Ada's Honda and head across the I-90 bridge to the Bellevue Red Lion to Amma's temporary lair. The parking lot is filled with thousands of cars belonging to people who have converged at the hotel to bask in the glory of their living goddess. Overwhelmed by the crowd (and the long distance from our parked car to the hotel entrance), I grab my purse and a cane I brought to stabilize my wimbly wombly gait.

"How are you feeling?" Ada asks. "I need to sit down." She immediately finds someone to fetch a chair for me while we wait in the ticket line to get our hugs from Amma Mama. "Don't worry." Ada assures me, "You won't have to wait in the regular line. Sit down, I'll be right back."

I initally felt slightly sheepish bringing a cane I don't normally use, but Ada warned me that the wait to get a hug can be up to eight hours — and dey ain't no way I can stand — nor sit — that long without some additional support.

She returns with someone wearing a long flowing silk scarf and they usher me into the hotel's large exhibition hall packed with devotees, many in white dresses and pants creating a feeling that this is really — *an event*. Ada and the long-scarf lady inform me they're taking me to the "Assisted" hug area, making it sound like I'm on my way to the "Special Bus" section of this ride. I hobble, lean on my cane as we flow through the enormous sea of white — then someone calls out.

"Deirdre?!?" a woman says, looking at my cane and reaching out to hug me. "How are you?"

"Great," I hug back with no idea who this person is. "But you know ..." I peter off, looking at the cane.

"Oh, I am so sorry," she says earnestly. "I heard. How are you do-ing?"

"Fine, just, gettin' through it. Hoping Amma can cure my brain cancer."

"Yeah, she will," the woman says.

"Yeah, she will," I repeat, nodding in agreement. "Okaaay, well, I gotta sit down."

"Oh! Of course!" she says, glancing at the cane again.

"Well, have a nice hug," I tell her.

"You too, Deirdre. Have a nice hug," she says, all-knowingly.

"Who was that?" asks Ada.

"I have no idea," I tell her. "Not only can I not skip, I cannot remember a damn thing."

After waiting a while, our seats are reserved for us, and we're free to wander our way through the hall, discovering the Amma 'market' — filled with booths hawking all kinds of holy knick-knacks like incense and pictures of the goddess.

"I wonder how much she makes at these events," I say to Ada.

"I don't know, I'm sure it's a lot. She tours all around the world. But proceeds go to charitable acts for things like disaster relief and orphanages." Ada replies.

"Hmmm," I say. My atheist background has programmed me to question all things religious or spiritual. It's challenging for me to overcome my cynical questioning.

"What?" Ada says.

"Did I say something out loud?" I ask her.

"No, I just see you judging it," she answers. "There are people of all and no faiths here. I don't really think of it as a religion. It's just about receiving and celebrating unconditional motherly love. Amma says her only religion is love."

"… that makes a lot of money on tchotchkes," I finish. "Sorry, Ada, these kinds of things bring out the skeptic in me."

"It's OK. I get it. She did make the largest single aid contribution for Hurricane Katrina. And she encourages her devotees to help and selflessly serve in their own communities to make it better. So to me, it ain't all so bad," she smiles. "Do you want to go sit back down?"

As we sit in the handicapped section (cane at my feet), we wait a couple of hours, slowly moving up through rows of chairs with each new round of believers that line up on stage.

Swathed in white fabric with a dot painted on her forehead, Amma sits in a puffy, silken throne trimmed with roses, surrounded by a throng of orange-robed assistants on a platform on stage. People file up to her one by one, getting down on their knees to be swallowed by her strong embrace. She rocks back and forth hugging each devotee, saying something in their ear, then hands them a packet of holy ash — (I've heard) blessed by the goddess — a Hershey's Kiss, and some flower petals.

"What's the chocolate kiss for?" I ask Ada, secretly wishing they were mini peanut butter cups.

"Amma always gives them. Reminds us there's always something sweet to look forward to in life," Ada says, getting quieter and eyes locking on Amma as we near the stage.

I think of a million jokes I want to crack, but remember I promised myself I would behave on this little adventure.

"Oh, that's sweet," I say, resisting the temptation to say, "Sweet. Get it? Get it?"

After four hours, our line has finally, finally, finally crept up to actually being on stage. I watch with fascination as people on stage cry and sway after hugging Amma. One woman is even speaking in tongue — or at least a tongue I've never heard before.

The hours of live chanting from a band behind Amma, the mass praying, the blur of people in white clothing milling around, the smell of rose incense, and the general intensity of the vibe in the huge exhibition hall has kind of put me under a spell. As my turn approaches, I gotta tell ya, I get a little bit caught up in it all and against my own smart-alecky self, I'm actually getting excited for my hug.

Ding, ding, ding. It's my turn. The hugger in front of me stands up.

The handlers direct me where and how to sit, and somebody reads Amma a note in Hindi. Apparently, you can pass notes to Amma, and translators will read them to her as you sit down for your hug. Well, Ada has forwarded such a note to Amma on my behalf telling her that I have brain cancer.

I take in *the goddess* — her dark skin, her long hair, her white robe, her forehead dot. Being as this is the first *goddess* I've ever met, I don't know what to expect. Will she glow? Or will her eyes be all pupil? Or will she be ever so slightly elevated off the ground? But, no. There's nothing I can glean that is extraordinary, she just looks like a really sweet old grandma sitting in her puffy, flowery silk armchair.

"Hi, Amma," I say.

Amma reaches to me and pulls me into her ample bosom, rocking back and forth and repeating, "My daughter. My daughter. My daughter." Then she hands me two (!) chocolates and two (!) packets of ash and hugs me AGAIN, this time handing me an apple!

I'm thinking I won the Amma lottery because she not only doubled up on my loot, but she hugged me and only me TWICE. And I got an apple. And the hug? It was soft but firm. And she smelled really good from a variety of Indian essences and something I swear I've smelled at Macy's.

But I have to admit, Amma's hug (and second hug!) is so pleasant, I feel like I could bask in this soft, gently swaying, sweet-smelling bosom for eternity.

Seemingly over before it began, Amma releases me from my hug. Someone helps me up, hands me my cane and directs me off stage and away from the warm embrace of serenity.

I smell my packets of ash, my chocolate kisses and my apple. They smell sweet and aromatic. When I look back at Amma, she is already on to her next hug.

And here I am, prostrate before you, to confess that… I was overwhelmed by the hug, tear-eyed and feeling that indeed, I had just been swathed in holy love.

A few weeks after the Amma hug, May 21st arrives, marking something that I thought I would never see happen again.

My birthday.

At first, I wanted to host a big shindig with balloons and maybe a band and a big-ass cake — just really put on the dog, go hog wild, swill champagne, and in general, honor the miracle of one more year. But as I talk about hosting a big party with Rose and Jack, just discussing said celebration exhausts me: the cleaning, the shopping, the decorating, the sending of invitations, the booking of a band, the 'all' of it. So I decide to forgo a huge affair and instead opt for a family dinner at a little Italian restaurant near Lake Union.

After a delicious dinner, we head back to our house for an after-dinner drink. I notice Jack goes through the back gate instead of the front door, which is odd, yet I don't think anything of it. Remember, I have chemo brain and not all of my pistons are working.

Jack leads me and several close family members around the corner of our house and into the garden, which is filled with friends, neighbors and loved ones all shouting, "SURPRISE!!!"

It was like getting love-bombed. I felt like I was being physically punched in the gut with love.

I lose it, bursting into tears. For the next hour, I sob on the shoulders of every single guest, hugging each person and being overwhelmed by the pulsating, palpable, heavenly hugs of everyone around me. And I believe each and every one of those hugs packs the same punch as an Amma hug. Because those hugs contain the magic ingredient of Amma's hugs. That's right. Love.

Proof of progress and hope for the future. The moments that mark the sweetness of life and reward for hard work. The denouement of childhood and the inauguration of adulthood. These are descending on Rose and her friends tonight as they attend their high school graduation.

In a ceremony of much pomp and circumstance, each graduate sits in a throne (literally, a *throne*) on stage while a slide show of their time at school plays on a screen behind them.

Affectionately calling her 'Rosemarian the Librarian' for her serious approach to her studies, Rosemary's teachers laud her accomplishments as a dedicated academic and an all-around nice person. Listening to the teachers go on about her high school career creates a dreamlike montage. Walking her to the park stooped over to hold her hand. Pushing her on the swing. Whooshing her down the slide. Making her favorite homemade chicken sticks and mac-and-cheese. Sitting on the bathroom floor splashing her tummy and giving her bubble-bath crowns. Holding her as she cries at the doctor's while getting the latest inoculation. Taking silly photos at the orthodontist as they stretch her mouth open to work on her teeth. Sitting by her side and holding her hand, which she squeezes as the dentist fills a cavity. Boiling oatmeal for breakfast and decorating it with a fruit face. Packing lunch — PB&J, fruit, yogurt. Escorting her to dance class. Scrambling to find her tennis and soccer games. Making her laugh. Making her laugh even harder. Sneaking sleepovers with her in bed. Bandaging her boo-boos. Taking her to the zoo and to Nana's and to school. Watching "Sleeping Beauty" over and over (and over). Reading "Harry Potter" out loud in her big-girl bed. Hugging her when she meets me at the gate after school and kissing her when she falls.

The memories wash over me as Rose majestically sits on stage, smiling while her teachers call out her successes. Her happiness is worth everything to me, and I thank Gaia for letting me live to this moment.

I've decided Rose is a Rolling Stone. In the time I've been in treatment, she has danced at prom, traveled to England, graduated high school, and soon she will spend the summer trekking in China with money she's saved from her weekend job in a coffee shop.

Though I now feel gratefully confident that I will continue to share a life with Rose, I also feel gratefully confident that Rose will be able to kick some mighty ass, with or without me. She has blossomed into a competent young woman perfectly capable of maneuvering life's challenges. She is … an adult.

Just days after graduation, Rose starts to lay out clothing, boots, hats, Tampax, toothbrush, dry shampoo, wet shampoo, sleeping bag — everything she'll need for trekking in China for the summer. Stuffing a huge hiking backpack for her journey, we double and triplecheck that she has her passport, her visa, her phone, her safety essentials for her six-week trip in various regions of China, starting in Beijing where she will meet her boyfriend Saul.

Once again, Jack and I stand outside the airport security line and dab our eyes as our little gazelle takes off her shoes, removes her electronics and passes through airport security.

"*Sayonara!*" I yell.

"That's Japanese," Jack says.

"Oh, right. *Ciao!*" I yell as she clears security.

"Italian," Jack corrects.

"*Au revoir? Adios? Auf Wiedersehen?*"

"French. Spanish. German," he says.

"Bye!" I say, giving, Jack the skunk eye.

Rose waves her hand as she walks out of sight.

"Come on," he takes my arm. "You have a chemo appointment."

My visit to Candyland has been a far longer trip than I somehow expected and although I'm thankful to still be alive, I'm ready to get off this game board.

"Hello Deirdre," says my oncologist as he follows me and Jack into my patient room at the clinic. "Your blood counts are still low, but I believe by next week they'll be high enough for another round," he tells me. It's June and coming on more than two months since my last infusion, which I'm supposed to get every six weeks. But my white blood cell count lingers around 2, and the doctor won't proceed until it reaches a minimum count of 5.

"As far as your chemo is concerned, I think your body is ready to quit. Your blood has been flagging through the whole process. I think we can end treatment after your next treatment, which would be your fourth treatment."

"Wait, let me digest this," I tell him, putting my coat back on after a hot flash. "If we end treatment early, am I at greater risk for the cancer spreading?"

"There's no way of knowing," he says. "What we do know is that your body is not recuperating quickly enough between treatments. Part of the effectiveness of chemo is regular and frequent infusions. If it's months between each treatment, it's not nearly as effective, if at all. I believe your body is finished with this."

It's ending? This will all be over soon? I just hadn't planned for this news. On the one hand, nothing sounds better than an end to this folly. On the other hand, I feel like I failed Chemo 101 and now my future health might be compromised because I couldn't finish.

"Well? What do you think?" he asks.

I look at Jack. I can't read what he's thinking.

"Jack?" I query. "What do you think?"

"I don't know, honey," he responds. "If your body can't take any-more, that seems to answer the question."

I look at the doctor.

"Alright," I say. "Let's end this game."

Three days later, Jack calls up the stairs. "I'm in the car!"

"Wait!" I yell down. "Just let me grab my computer." I unplug my MacBook Air and descend. I'm wearing a blue knit dress and leggings — 'chemo clothes' — something that's comfortable enough to lie in bed for hours.

"You look cute," Jack remembers to tell me. I don't look cute, but it's nice to hear. I look tired. My hair is growing in for a second time, but other hair is still falling out. It's a curious dichotomy. I don't even bother to draw on fake eyebrows and paint lipstick on my pale lips.

"Thank you," I say.

"Do you have everything?" he asks. "Is your phone charged?

"I can charge it at the hospital," I tell him.

"Nervous?" he asks.

"Yeah, kind of," I start to tear up. "It's all been so random. This whole past year. Fuck."

"Well, hopefully it ends today and life can return to normal," he says, hugging me.

"No shit," I say. "That sounds nicer than nice."

We drive to the hospital in silence, park, take the elevator to the third floor and walk to the blood draw unit. The needle poke hurts and the phlebotomist has to work hard to hit a healthy vein several times. Then we ascend to the chemo unit on the eighth floor.

"What's a girl gotta do to get some chemo around here?" I joke with the techs.

"Deirdre, how are you?" they ask in unison.

"This is my last chemo session," I smile. "I know you're gonna miss me, but things have to end between us. Don't worry … it's not you, it's me."

"Congratulations," my nurse says. "That's great news! Come on, let's get you going so you can get out of here and hopefully, never come back!"

"Amen," I say.

We go through the rigamarole: Start an IV drip of saline, wait for the orders from the blood lab that I'm good to go, order the chemo, set the chemo infusion, wait, sleep, look out the window, ponder.

"Do you want me to stay?" Jack asks.

"No, it's going to be six hours," I tell him. "Just come back around 4."

"OK honey," he says, bending down to kiss me. "Congratulations. We can have champagne tonight."

"I think that's totally in order!"

For six hours, I absorb lyrics on Pandora rather than crack open my computer. The time passes quickly, and before I know it, I'm driving home from my final chemo treatment. I feel an exhilarating sense of ease. It's a beautiful June day, just like the day I received my terminal diagnosis exactly one year ago. Summer is in full swing. It's sunny. Trees are in bloom and children skip down the sidewalk. The world looks so beautiful.

Only now, I don't see the panorama through a filter of finality. I'm not taking things in with the feeling of disappearance — looping on the same ongoing questions of *Will I ever drive down this street again?* or *Will I outlive that ladybug?* or *How long before I am just that distant dusty memory?* Instead, I pass neighborhoods I know so well — Capitol Hill, the Central District, Leschi and Madrona, with an excited sense of calm relief. *We'll have to try that new restaurant*, I think, passing a new

Thai place on Cherry. *Look at that yard, it's gorgeous. I'll have to renovate my long-neglected yard. Where do I want to have dinner tonight?*

Taking deep breaths, I inhale life — without fear that every experience, every conversation and every meal may be my last.

I take off my jacket and open the car window. Another hot flash burns through my body and drenches my dress. I stick my head out of the window like a dog craving the cooling wind of speed. It smells like exhaust and jasmine. I'm even thankful for the whiff of pollution because it's sensual proof that I am a living part of this human tribe.

I plot the rest of my first day back. I'll walk the dogs — not far — I'm still too weak. But farther than I have been. Maybe I'll shoot for three blocks.

I'll make a JibJab for Rosie, who safely arrived in China with her boyfriend Saul. She turns 18 today and I can't help but think that it's somehow prophetic that I'm completing treatment on the day of her birth. I feel like we now share a birthday. In a Hallmark way, this feels like the first day of the rest of my life.

Nagging hunger interrupts my thoughts. The steroids still have a grip on my appetite.

"Can we stop at Naam?" I ask Jack. Naam is my favorite Thai place four blocks from my house.

"Sure," he says, rushing through a yellow light.

Exhaling, I close my window and put my jacket back on. Just like all of my hot flashes, this one is followed by a bone-chilling cold flash. I turn my seat-warmer on and tighten my jacket around my neck, even though it's 72 degrees outside.

As we park next to the restaurant, I wait for Jack to open my door and lend me a hand as I weakly hoist out of the car. Some *pad see ew* should quell my grumbling stomach. Three stars. And fresh rolls. And thick sweet Thai ice tea. If they have sticky rice with mango and coconut milk, I'm even going to order dessert.

And then, I plan to nestle in bed with my two dogs … and sleep and sleep and sleep and sleep.

𝄠 𝄠 𝄠

Jack wakes me up the next morning while getting ready to go to his evolving restaurant.

"Good morning," he smiles when he sees me open my eyes. "How'd you sleep?"

"Oh God, I kept waking up. Hot. Cold. Hot. Cold. This chemo-induced menopause is a bitch. But that's OK cuz it makes me so sexy with a thick waist and thin hair and a shriveled va-jay-jay," I smile.

"Cut yourself some slack," he tells me.

"Knock knock."

"Who's there?" he plays along.

"Your wife."

"Your wife who?"

"Your wife, who's still here," I joke. "Now, give me a kiss and go to work. I have some serious resting to do."

"Love you," he says, bending down to kiss me.

"Me too," I tell him. "I mean, I love you too. Not I love me too."

"Yeah yeah," he says, turning at the door. "I'm glad you're alive."

As I hear his feet hit the stair treads, my nose starts to run and my eyes start to water.

Thirteen months ago, I had no idea that just waking up in bed would be such a relief.

CHAPTER 21

The third floor

More often than not these days, when I show up at the home for dementia and Alzheimer's patients, Kathy is asleep. And when I say she's "asleep," I mean that she is so deep in slumber and there is no waking her.

"Mom, hi!" I say, kissing her on the cheek. "Mom, can you wake up? Mooommm, wake up. D-D's here."

Nothing. She's seated in a wheelchair.

"Is she on different drugs?" I ask the nurse.

"No, they're all the same," she tells me.

Kathy's on a pill wagon with bulging sides, taking meds for everything from pain (arthritic hip), to Alzheimer's, to anxiety, to diarrhea, to constipation, to general health, to sleep, you name it. Throughout the day she swallows Vitamin D3; Culturelle, Quetiapine, Meloxicam, Metamucil, Citalopram and Senna-Gen. She's now barely able to chew and swallow, so her pills take a while to get down aided by sips of juice.

As Kathy pulls out of her unconscious state, she smiles but says nothing. Then, her face distorts as she throws her head back.

"OH GOD IN HEAVEN, STOP THIS PAIN," she screams. "AAAAAGHH! HELP ME! HELP ME!"

I grab the nurse.

"What's going on?! What can we do?!" I implore. "This is not OK!"

"I'll get her something to kill the pain," she says.

As Kathy screams and cries out for mercy, I watch the door. What is taking the nurse so long? After what feels like a lifetime, the nurse enters with a small paper cup containing pink liquid.

"Here you go, Kathy. Open up. This is to stop your pain. Come on honey, open up."

In between screams, the nurse tries to pour the pink goo into her mouth, most of which pours out of Kathy's mouth and down her chin. I run my fingers through her curly hair and tell her everything's gonna be OK and the meds just have to take effect.

After several more minutes of crying out, Kathy stops screaming and her head slumps once again.

"Can you see to it that the doctor takes a look at Kathy?" I ask. "I mean this is a nightmare. I've never seen her in so much pain."

"Actually, your mom has an appointment tomorrow," the nurse tells me.

"OK, I'll come back tomorrow to check in," I tell her. "Call me if anything changes. You know I can be here in 15 minutes."

"We will," the nurse assures me.

I look down at my mother. Her skin is gray. Food covers her shirt. Her mouth is slack. She's fading. I can see it. Why haven't I made it here more often? I kick myself. What have I let happen to you, Mom? I'm so sorry. I've failed you.

Hugging my mother, I kiss her on the forehead and leave.

The next day I return to the nursing home.

Again, Kathy is deep in sleep.

"Mom, wake up," I urge. "It's D-D your daughter. Wake up! I brought you a cookie."

She doesn't budge. If her chest didn't rise and fall, I'd think she was dead.

"Has she been like this since yesterday?" I ask a nurse.

"She's just napping. She's awake most of the night lately."

"Napping?" I say. "She's catatonic."

"Deirdre," somebody says behind me. It's Hannah, the home's director.

We exchange hugs and I ask her if my mom's meds have changed and how long she's been like this. Just a week ago, she was cracking jokes.

"I need to talk to you," she says, her eyes wide with sympathy. "Do you have time now?"

"Sure," I say, thinking, *This doesn't sound like a happy talk. I don't think I want to have this talk.*

"Sit down," she says as we head into her office. "Would you like some coffee or tea?"

"No thank you Hannah," I say, locking eyes with her. "You're about to make me cry, aren't you?"

"Well … your mother's doing fine, don't worry."

"Fine?" I ask rhetorically. "She's become a zombie. And when she does come out of this, this, this whatever — sleep — she's screaming in pain."

"The doctor increased her pain meds today, so it's natural that she's sleeping a lot. But Deirdre," she continues, "your mother is awake most nights and requires one-on-one attention. The only problem is, we're on a skeleton staff at night. However, on the third floor we are fully staffed 24/7."

"You want to move her to the third floor?" I ask, tearing up. "The third floor's the last floor."

"It's not all bad," she comforts me, handing me a tissue. "It's very quiet and sunny up there. The staff are wonderful. She can still come downstairs during the day and be with everyone here."

"When do you want to move her?" I choke.

"As soon as possible," she says. "An apartment has just come available. It's a shared apartment, so she'll have a roommate. Her roommate is a lovely woman and very quiet. Would you like to see it?"

"No, but yes," I tell her. I know I'm about to see the last bedroom my mother will ever sleep in.

As we ascend to the third floor, the elevator door opens to a sunny room, just as Hannah promised. A handful of residents sit in wheelchairs, sleeping. One lady is calling out for help, over and over again. A gentleman that I recognize from downstairs looks through me. He's 'graduated' to the third floor as well.

"This is the apartment," says Hannah walking me into a corner space. The nurse is helping my mom's future roommate on the toilet.

As the nurse sees us enter, she closes the door behind her. "And this would be your mother's bedroom."

It's not actually a bedroom. It's the apartment's original 'living room.' There's no closet and it's just … not a bedroom. Suddenly, it seems so important to me that she has a bedroom in which to retire to eternity.

"Do you have any single rooms?" I ask.

"Unfortunately, I don't," she tells me.

"Well, is anyone close to — you know — checking out soon?"

"Uhhhh, OK. There is one patient who may be leaving soon, if you catch my drift."

"I catch your drift. May I see that room?"

"Certainly."

The room is empty. While it doesn't have much of a view and it seems dark to me, it's leagues better than the other room. I can easily spruce this one up.

"The resident is currently in the hospital," Hannah tells me.

"This would be so much better," I tell her relieved. "Do you mind if we just wait until the current resident, um, moves on?"

"Certainly," she says. "I'd be happy to reserve the room for Kathy."

When I go downstairs, I see they've moved my mother to bed. I crawl under the covers and spoon her.

"Hi, Mom. You feel cozy in bed. This is much better than snoozing in a metal wheelchair."

"Love-a love-a love-a love-a love-a love-a love-a love-a love-a," she babbles.

"I love you too, Mom," I whisper. "I love you too."

🍭 🍭 🍭

Thanks to a year on steroids, I am no longer a bag of bones. In fact, quite the opposite — I weigh about what I weighed after giving birth to Rose. And because I like being thin better than anything on earth, this irritates me. As I struggle to button my "fat jeans," I try to tuck my flabby gut and swollen muffin top into the waist of my pants.

Dressing my ever-girthsome body triggers a hot flash, so I open the bedroom window and stick my head out to pant. As someone walks by the house, I sink to my knees so they won't see me in all my topless flubby glory. As they pass, I wrestle to stand up, clawing up the side of my bed like a ladder. I think of all the times I watched my obese father labor to stand up and how my own physical struggles remind me of him.

It's going to be in the 80s today — and with my hot flash still raging — I think maybe, just maybe, I can wear summery shoes instead of the snow boots that I've been wearing for the past 12 months. I slide my feet into my comfortable flip-flops, but as I take a step, the right flip-flop flies off my foot. *Odd*, I think. I put it back on, take a step, and it flies off again. I look down at the shoe, thinking the strap must be broken. It's not ... it's just that my right foot no longer has the coordination to grip a flip-flop.

Fine. I have a backup plan. I'll just wear my Tom's. I hold on to the wall for support as I bend over to slide on each fabric shoe. Then guess what? I take a step and the right Tom falls off. And I'm thinking, *Really? My foot can't hold on to a Tom? REALLY?* And, pardon my French, but again I'm like, *Fuck*!

I grab a sweatshirt and sit on my bed, still topless. My joints — particularly my shoulders — ache, I suppose from the radiation. I fight the pain to raise my arms above my head and slip on the ugliest, oldest, most paint-splattered sweatshirt in the world. Now that my hot flash has passed, I'm getting a chill.

I look at my winter boots. Alright, you win. Shivering, I shove each foot into my well-worn rubber Sorels and struggle to tie the laces.

I head downstairs, gripping the railing with each step and opening the doors to one very excited 65-pound ginger doodle. It doesn't matter to him that I only walk him a few yards before turning back to the house. It doesn't matter to him that I look like a homeless person. It doesn't matter to him that I'm not getting anything done. It just matters to him that I'm here, telling him he's a good boy and running my fingers through his bushy mane.

"Well, Arthur," I assure him, "This is it. We really need to start walking for realsies and get this flabalanche back in shape!"

BARK! BARK BARK BARK!

He's happy with this news.

I strap on his leash and head out the door, vowing to walk a few blocks more than I have been.

While walking I think about the other areas of my life I need to address. After a year of sitting in my living room and avoiding any and all participation in the real world, I have a lot of catching up to do. My house looks like a hoarder lives here — paperwork is piled on every ledge and table, dog hair floats around like ginger bunnies, my yard is overrun with blackberry bushes and dandelions — it's all just a mess. Rose is still trekking through China for the fourth week, but she'll be back in two weeks and I want to get the house and yard back into shape before she returns. I want to give her the sense that everything's just fine as wine.

Arthur hasn't seen a vet or had his teeth cleaned in a couple of years. He is long overdue for some medical attention. He smells like yeasty rotten vegetables from neglected teeth and ear infections. I've hardly visited the restaurant and Jack wants me to be there so I can help him with aesthetic decisions. As the quasi interior designer, I'm supposed to help formulate a look and feel for the space, which is quickly transforming from a demolition zone into a recognizable set of dining rooms with painted walls and a new kitchen. Though I'm no interior decorator, I'm a damn sight better at sprucing up a room than Jack. Left to his own devises, cardboard boxes covered with blankets would suffice as side tables and "art" would consist of pictures cut out from magazines and taped to the walls. I at least have a basic understanding of creating a homey entrance with our old IKEA sectional and sourcing recycled wooden dining chairs to create a country bohemian atmosphere.

After leaving Jack's one day, I swing onto the freeway entrance ramp that will take me to Kathy's. Now confined to her wheelchair because the pain of standing finally eclipsed her ability to ambulate, she floats in and out of consciousness. I feel her loneliness, her confusion — and her imminent demise — with every molecule of my existence and the pull to stay by her side is strong.

Jack calls while I'm with Kathy.

"Hey hon, what's up?" I ask him.

"A beam just fell on my foot," he tells me. "I gotta come home. It hurts like a motherfucker."

"Oh sweetie, I'm sorry," I sympathize. "I'll meet you at home."

"OK," he says. "See you in a sec."

I kiss Kathy and drive home. When Jack walks in the door, he's limping.

"Let's see it," I say, curious.

As he gingerly pulls off his shoe and sock, the largest purple-ist most blistered Big Bumble Boy I have ever seen wags at me.

"Yeowtch? How'd it happen?" I ask.

"One of the construction workers dropped this four by six beam and it clipped my foot."

"We should ice it," I advise. "And maybe take some ibuprofin?"

"I've been doing that. Nothing's helped," he says. "I'm just going to go to bed and keep it elevated. Fuck it hurts."

"OK. I'll bring up a bag of frozen peas to lay on it."

By morning, the toe is even larger, more blistered, and the purple is now deepened with red.

"I have to go to the emergency room. This is not OK," Jack says. "Can you drive me there?"

"Of course! Yes," I say enthusiastically. But really, I don't want to go back to a hospital. One of my great joys these past couple of weeks is the complete absence of medical facilities. No more hobbling around to endless appointments, getting poked and prodded and subjected to constant MRIs and CAT scans. That is, until now.

As we walk through the automatic door, I want to gag. The smell and sounds and atmosphere of the hospital are all too unpleasantly familiar. After seeing the nurse and then the doctor, Jack is rolled away in a wheelchair for an X-ray. Ugh, I think, secretly glad it's him not me.

When the tech wheels him back in, he tells Jack, "You did a doozie on that toe."

"You're going to have to have surgery," the doctor says after entering and pulling up the X-ray on the computer. "You have essentially crushed your toe. See how all of these bones are splintered? It will not repair on its own. Hopefully, we'll be able to save the toe."

"Shit," is Jack's first response. "'Save the toe?' It's that bad?"

"It's pretty bad," the doctor confirms.

"I don't have time for surgery. I'm opening a restaurant soon. I need all my toes."

"Sorry, buddy," the doctor apologizes. "The surgeon will probably be able to pin it together, but it is seriously injured. Surgery is your only option. I've scheduled you to meet with an excellent foot surgeon after this appointment. It's in the Nordstrom Tower. Do you know where that is?"

"I do," I say. "I know it well."

"Oh, baby," Jack says, holding onto my arm as he limps back to the car. "I'm so sorry to bring you back to a hospital. You just got out of all this. I am just so sorry."

"Honey, I don't care," I lie. "I just want you to get better."

The surgeon schedules his surgery for the next morning, sending us home with painkillers and instructions not to eat or drink anything after midnight.

When we get home Jack asks me, "Is it too early for a martini?"

"Under the circumstances, I think a three-martini lunch is perfectly appropriate."

The operation goes off without a hitch. While Jack's foot heals, I will have to be his driver. I note the irony that a year ago he had to be my driver, and now I have to be his. We pull up to his restaurant, his leg in a cast, Jack grabs his brand spankin' new crutches and limps to his future.

☺ ☺ ☺

"Let's get away," Jack suggests. Our 25th anniversary is next week. "Why don't we go to Victoria, where we had our first really romantic adventure?"

I don't want to travel. I want to wallow in my post-treatment fatigue, follow Rosemary's Chinese adventures on Facebook, and hang out with my mom. But, I figure, a trip might be a good thing to jump-start my recuperation. And since one of my primary goals is to become physically connected to Jack again — not a slug on a couch — I agree.

"OK. Yes. Yes, that's a good idea. We can celebrate our anniversary where it all began. Yes."

"I'll book it. I'm excited!" Jack tells me.

"Me too, Baby," I say. "But, do you mind if we don't go for long? I'm worried about leaving my mom."

"Just for the weekend," he promises.

One week later, we arrive at The Victoria Clipper dock on Seattle's waterfront. The boat is a cross between a small ferry and a small cruise ship. Because it has open seating, there's a long line of travelers who get there early to snag plum seats. When I see the line, I hide my disappointment. Standing for long periods of time makes me dizzy and flu-ish.

"Honey, do you mind if I sit while you check us in?" I ask, scanning the room for a place to plunk down.

"No no. Go sit over there. I'll flag you if you need to check in."

"Thanks."

He checks us in, though I have to present myself at the counter with my passport so they know Jack's not trying to sneak a terrorist or an illegal alien on board. Then, we join a line that wraps around the waterfront building. After what seems like ten years of standing and waiting in the line — taking my jacket off, stepping side-to-side, and putting my jacket back on — we board. The ride is beautiful — but I'm disappointed because the last time I took this boat 30 years ago, whales swam alongside the ship. Today, the waters are clear and still.

After settling into our hotel, we walk through the neighborhood, admiring the British-style gardens bursting in a gaudy display of geraniums, azaleas and rhododendrons. We roam the European-style waterfront town, lamenting the disappearance of the cheesy Madame Tussaud's Wax Museum, and peruse the Viking exhibit at one of the museums.

"Okaaaay," Jack says, eyes at half mast. "That put me to sleep. Wanna get a beer?"

"I don't know. I could take a second trip around the warrior exhibit," I kid.

We head into the street and pick one of the many Irish pubs with seemingly pre-pubescent girls waiting tables in micro-mini plaid skirts.

"This one?" Jack asks.

"Sure, whatever. I just want to sit down."

As Jack watches the beautiful girls, I sulk over my beer feeling like a wet clump of clay stuffed with poo-brains.

"You wanna take a nap?" he asks, sensing my complete lack of enjoyment. In fact, no, I'm like a black hole of enjoyment, sucking in every atom of happiness around me.

"Sure. Whatever." Then I chide myself for being a killjoy on the first purely romantic holiday Jack and I have shared in many years. "That was fun," I lie.

"Those girls were so cute," he says, not in a dirty-old-man way but just calling out the truth.

"I know, right?!" I say with a smile, shooting daggers in my mind. "They remind me of Rose, your daughter."

"Yeah, totally," he says, oblivious to my resentful fake-happy voice. "It's good to be young."

As I huff and puff up the small hill, I think, *It is good to be young. But when you're young you don't know how good it is to be young. You only appreciate it in retrospect.*

"Yup. Good to be young," I agree, with another beaming faux smile.

After an epic nap, I shake off my resentment at not being 20 and tan and tiny in a mini-plaid skirt. Jack's made reservations at a French restaurant where we had our first fancy meal together. As we arrive, they have a romantic table set with flowers for our anniversary.

"You've remodeled," I tell the waiter. "But then, the last time we were here was 26 years ago."

"Oh, no we have not remodeled," corrects the waiter. "In fact, we opened fairly recently."

"No, because we celebrated our love here in the '80s," Jack informs him. "The owner was Jean something …"

"You're thinking of *Sur La Mer* in Vancouver, I believe," suggests the waiter.

"Wait. No. What?" burps Jack.

"Oui. Sur La Mer. It was in Vancouver," he says, refilling our champagne glasses before turning on his heels and returning to the kitchen.

Jack and I look at each other.

"Wasn't it Victoria we came to all these years ago?" he asks me.

"You know what?" I question. "It WAS Vancouver. We're in the wrong city! We came here with your mother all those years ago and it wasn't romantic … it was boring!"

"I can't believe I confused the two cities," Jack marvels.

"Now who has the broken brain?" I tease him.

"Yeah right?!" he laughs. "Sheesh. We're quite the pair."

Secretly, I'm pleased that Jack confused the memory. I'm so tired of being the only one who is lost in time and space, and I have to admit, it's nice having someone else slip up.

I visit my mom once we return to Seattle. She's sleeping in her wheelchair in the same place and in the same room as when I visited her a few days ago. It's as if I left her for five minutes and came right back to her. She is frozen in her own life. Time passes, but she doesn't.

"Mom, wake up," I nudge her shoulder. "Wake up. Deirdre your daughter is here."

I stare at her, drinking her in. I think about what a lousy cook she was except for the Sunday morning waffles she executed flawlessly every weekend to my and Sam's great delight. I think about the boxing gloves she bought me and Sam so when we got in fights, we could put them on and not hurt each other (as much). I think about how she would get in tickling matches with me and Sam on the couch in the family room, eliciting squeals of joy from us. I think of how fiercely she defended us against anything — neighborhood bullies, judgmental socialites, and critical teachers. I think about how we could do no wrong in her eyes (but if we did, boy did she let us have it). I think about just how funny and honest and eccentric she was — a genuine original with her fuzzy fly-away hair and a complete disinterest in "fitting in." I think about what a loving, generous — and at times scary — person she was, and yet she was always my best friend, my loving mother and my ultimate supporter. And now, here she sits before me, slumped over, unable to speak or eat — and I'm guessing soon — unable to breathe.

After many minutes, she lifts her lids and looks past me.

"Hi!" I bubble. Today I closed on her house. I debate telling her, but decide not to. The truth is, I feel a little sheepish about selling her home. I know there's not a chance in hell that she'll ever return, but still, I feel like I sold it out from under her. She had always told me, "When I go, you can have the house. Or maybe Rose can have it. Wouldn't that be great?" But the economics of holding on to a second home didn't make sense and all of her kids already owned homes.

"Hell," she says.

"Hell, or hello?" I ask.

"Hello," she corrects herself.

"Probably a little bit of Hell thrown in there too," I say, kissing her on the cheek. "Sooooo, how ya doin?"

"Fie," she mumbles very quietly while looking through me.

"I'm fine too," I smile, hoping she'll catch my smile. "Jack and I went to Victoria this weekend."

No response.

"Rosie's still in China. But she'll be home in less than two weeks. Won't that be fun to see her?"

"Mmmm," she replies.

"Look, I brought you a Reese's," I say. Reese's have been her crack since I was a kid. "Here, take a bite." She doesn't move a muscle, so I try to manipulate her mouth open. "Here mom, Reese's."

I finally get a bite in her. She doesn't chew it. She doesn't swallow it. She just leaves her mouth half-open with the chocolate melting on her tongue. A nurse walks up and bends over Kathy, speaking very clearly into her ear.

"Kathy, it's time for your afternoon meds," she tells her.

"Um, she has a bite of candy bar in her mouth," I tell the nurse. "She won't be able to take pills with that sitting in there."

"Oh. Kathy, swallow your bite. If you can't swallow it, you can spit it out," she says, reaching into her mouth and removing 'the obstruction.' "OK, here you go."

She pops a few pills into my mom's mouth and pours orange drink into her mouth, closing Kathy's mouth and tipping her head back and instructing her to swallow.

"OK, open up," instructs the nurse. "Good job, Kathy. We got 'em down."

"Hey, I have a question," I interrupt the nurse as she turns to tend to the next patient. "How long has she not been eating?"

"She's eating," the nurse assures me. "Sometimes she just needs encouragement with a sip of something between each bite."

I know with Alzheimer's one of the final stages of the disease is the inability to eat. Feeding tubes are not an option because at this advanced stage, the body can no longer 'remember' how to digest food. I've read that oftentimes Alzheimer's patients actually starve to death because they can no longer take in nutrition, and I wonder, *Is this just a phase or is this … it?*

"D-D," my mom manages. Oh good, she's back. I'll try some light banter to see if she can join me.

"I've been working on my garden. You taught me how to garden. You always had such beautiful gardens, Mom," I tell her. "It's kind of challenging for me. You know I can't bend over 'cuz of my weakness and balance issues from treatment. Remember? I have cancer."

Kathy groans.

"Oh, but it's OK, they cured it," I reassure her so she doesn't get upset. "Anyway, while I'm gardening I sit on the ground and scootch around to pick weeds and clip branches. My butt gets completely dirty. But it's nice to have my hands in the soil and sit in the sun and see the improvement. You know I don't think I've worked in my yard in years."

"Mmmm," she repeats, still looking through me.

"Want to see a picture of my garden?" I ask her.

"Mmmm."

"Here it is," I say, holding up my iPhone with a photo of Butchart Gardens — one of the world's most beautiful gardens in Victoria, B.C. "Pretty nice, huh?"

"It's OK, I guess," she says, uttering a full sentence.

"OK?! It's ..." I start. But I stop mid-sentence. She got me.

After squeezing out a joke, my mom immediately returns to deep slumber.

CHAPTER 22

Until we meet again

We're getting dangerously close to opening the restaurant. Originally, we thought we'd be open by June 1. That didn't happen. Renovating the run-down space has been a game of sorting out plumbing, electrical and structural nightmares. As each new roadblock gets smoothed out, we announce the soft opening for Aug. 1. But as problems continue to surface (and several break-ins), that day came and went. It's now Aug. 6 and we're telling people — for sure — the doors will open on Sept. 1.

As I'm driving to the restaurant with napkins, to-go boxes, candleholders and salt-and-pepper shakers, my cell rings. It's my mom's nursing home. I do a quick scan for cops then answer the phone.

"Howdy doody," I answer, belying my hesitation.

"Deirdre, hello it's Hannah," says the director. "How are you?"

"Fine, what's up?" I ask her.

"Well, we are concerned about your mother," she responds. "She is struggling and we're not quite sure which direction to go with her. I think it would be best if you come — right away. Is that possible?"

"I'll be there in 10," I tell her.

I pull over to the side of the road. I think of all the times my mother sang "You Are My Sunshine" to us (off key, very off key, it sounded more like "Edelweiss" from "The Sound of Music") ... and I hold my head and I cry. I know on some instinctual level that this is the final call I've been dreading.

After snorting down snot and licking my tears, I head away from the restaurant — toward Mercer Island and my mother. As I walk up the stairs and enter the nursing home lobby, the staff give me sympathetic smiles.

"How are you, Deirdre?" Janice, the receptionist asks.

"Fine, but you know," I say, tearing up again, "Kathy."

She stands and gives me a hug as Hannah comes out of her office.

"Deirdre, hello," she says, also taking me in her arms. "Shall we go up and visit your mother or do you want to take a moment?"

"No, let's go."

My mom's in bed, babbling gibberish. I climb in bed with her and hold her. She starts to scream in anguish.

"Isn't there something we can give her for pain?" I plea to Hannah. "Morphine? Anything?"

"Well, we have a decision to make," Hannah informs me. "We need to decide whether to take her to the hospital ..."

"No, no no no no," I say. "That's the last place she should be. They'll just poke and prod her and check on her all night so she can't rest and for what? Are they really gonna stop what's happening now? I mean ..." I burst out crying, unable to finish my sentence.

"There is the slight possibility that she has a secondary infection that has put her in this state," Hannah reasons. "If she does and

319

they're able to treat it with IV fluids and antibiotics, she just might recuperate."

"So, you think I should take her to the hospital?" I ask, wanting someone else to make this decision for me.

"It's up to you."

I look at my mother, who's writhing in pain and calling out with screams. *But what if,* I think, *what if this is just another urinary tract infection that's kicked her into this hellacious state?*

"Let's call the ambulance," I tell her.

As I wait for the medics to arrive, I call Jack and tell him what's happening. Then I call my brother Sam, who lives in Albuquerque.

"Hey, D-D," he answers.

"Sam," I say, trying my damnedest to hold it together. "I think Mom is … at the end."

"You always say that," he answers.

"No, this is different," I tell him. "I think she's actively dying. I'm waiting for the medics to come get her and take her to Swedish. I think you should come home now."

"I can't," he tells me. "Work is a shit-show right now."

"Sam, I don't think you have a choice," I press on. "She's no longer eating or responding. I think this is it."

"Tell you what, when you get to the hospital, let me know what the doctors say," he reasons with the comfort of distance. "I'll look at flights. But if this is temporary, I can't really leave work."

"It is temporary," I assure him. "Very temporary. She's dying."

As I follow the ambulance, I start calling others … my half-brother Don who has a different mother but grew up with my mom, and my cousin Ada. "Maybe you can stop by the hospital today? I can text you when I find out where we're gonna be."

They all agree to swing by after work.

I call Rosemary, who's still in China. Miraculously, she answers.

"Honey, Nana's not doing well," I tell her. "I think she's dying."

"Oh, Mom, I'm so sorry," she says. "Should I come home now?"

"No," I tell her. "You'll be home in four days. I think she'll last that long. But, just, I don't know, send her your prayers and be prepared for a sad homecoming."

"Are you sure you don't want me to come home now?" she asks.

The truth is, I don't want Rose to see her grandmother suffering and screaming out in anguish. It's just too horrific.

As they lift Kathy onto the gurney, she is still screaming and crying out. I smooth her kinky hair and hold her hand while doctors and nurses float in and out.

"Deirdre Timmons?" a doctor asks walking in.

"Yes," I answer.

"This is your mother?" he asks.

"Yes," I tell him.

"Your mother doesn't have a secondary infection," he tells me. "But she is severely dehydrated, so we're going to start giving her an IV with potassium and see if that brings her back."

"OK," I say.

"We'd like to move her upstairs into a private room for a night so we can keep an eye on her. Are you OK with that?"

"Yes," I tell him. "But … are they going to disturb her every half hour for vitals?"

"We'll do everything we can to keep her comfortable," he assures me.

"Is she … dying?" I ask.

"We don't know, only time will tell."

As I follow her through the web of hallways and elevators, keeping my hand on her foot so she's knows I'm with her, she continues to cry and moan.

"This is her room," says the tech, wheeling her into a room with a beautiful view of Capitol Hill. "Do you need anything else?"

"Can I have a fold-out chair or a cot to sleep with her tonight?" I ask.

"I'll ask the nurse," he says. "If it's not a problem I'll bring it right away."

"Thank you."

Several nurses and techs enter and introduce themselves. I tell them unless they have some life-saving care, I would just like the room to be as peaceful as possible while we receive family and friends. Nobody has said, "She's dying," to me, but I know she is. This is her last stop.

When we are alone, I close the door and shut the curtain at her door.

"Mom," I lean into her ear. "You've been one of the great loves of my life. I love you so much. But I think your time has come to let go and move on to the next stage, whatever that is. I have to ask you one last favor though. Can you please hold on until Sam and Rosie get here? It might take a couple of days, but they're trying to get here as quickly as possible."

She cries out.

"I'll be here with you for every second," I assure her. "I won't leave you until you're ready to leave me."

After a series of wrenching days and nights, I'm exhausted from no sleep. Kathy's cries have gone from screams of pain to calling out those who have passed before her.

"I don't wanna go, Mama!!!" she cries over and over again.

"No Daddy, don't make me go!!!" she yells.

She also calls out her siblings who have already left the earth: Carol! Richard! Virginia! Ed! (her brother in law).

It's unsettling how her cries are not calls of recognition and love. She seems to be begging everyone she's seeing not to make her go. *She doesn't wanna die,* I think. *She's scared.*

I try to assure her that it's all right, but then I think, *How presumptuous. Up until my cancer, I didn't even believe in life after death. Now I kind of do, but what if I'm wrong? What if something horrible awaits her — or what if it's just all-consuming blackness she sees and it's freaking her out? Whatever she's experiencing now, she doesn't like. My dad's death was so peaceful, but Kathy's death is so tortuous.*

I was with my father when he passed two years ago. It was one of the most intimate moments of my life. As he drew his final breaths, I told him how much he meant to me and kissed him on the forehead. We were alone in his nursing home. It was a warm October morning and the sun filtered into his room. As he emitted a final cough, I looked at him and said, "Dad, did you just die?" I watched his chest. It did not rise. I leaned in and whispered, "You can take another breath."

But he never did. For one, two, three minutes I concentrated on his chest. Realizing that he really had died, I collapsed over his body and hugged him, sobbing. I felt he was still in the room.

"I'll try to make you proud," I called to the room. "Thank you. Thank you for everything, Dad. Most of all, thank you for life."

"I'm here to take his vitals," a nurse said, bursting through the door.

"He has no vitals," I tell her, standing up. "He just died."

As I called family to come gather at his deathbed and wish him off to hopefully some wonderful magical existence, I felt honored to have shared his last breaths. It was as intimate as having a baby. The whole world felt so quiet ... and right. Watching my dad release into the Great Beyond was oddly beautiful. It was his time, and he left willingly.

It gave me a glimpse into the notion that we don't know (or many of us don't profess to know) where we come from and where we're headed ... but it doesn't seem like a bad place.

We keep Kathy on a saline drip in hopes of keeping her alive until Sam and Rose arrive. The fug of death permeates the room.

"What is that smell?" I ask the nurse, holding onto Kathy's hand.

"Her body has started to decompose," the nurse tells me. "I'll get you some ground coffee beans to absorb the smell. It might help."

"How can she start decomposing while she's still alive?" I ask, thinking immediately of salmon swimming upstream as their fins and faces rot and fall off, yet, they're still swimming.

"Sometimes it happens," she says. "It's not pleasant, but it's not unusual."

This is the single worst experience I've ever had in my life. It's far worse than the initial prognosis of my cancer.

Four days later my brother Sam arrives, causing me to breathe a deep sigh of relief. I haven't left the hospital or bathed in three nights. Though many friends (particularly childhood friends) have showed up and we've showered Kathy in love, laughing as we tell old stories about her hilarious antics and crying as we say goodbye, I need a break.

"Sam," I stand up, hugging him quickly before he moves on to Mom. "I'm so glad you made it."

"Hi, Kathy," he says into her ear. "It's Sam, your son. I'm here."

While he dotes on her, I excuse myself to go home and bathe.

"Sam, can you stay here tonight? I'm exhausted."

"Yeah, go on," he frees me.

"Mom, now that Sam is here, I'm going to go home and shower. I'll come back later," I say into her ear. "Mom, Rose will be here tomorrow. Can you hold on one more day? She loves you very much. You've been a big part of her life. Please hold on for one more day. I love you. Hold on." I turn to Sam. "OK, I'm leaving. If anything changes, call me. You know I live like five minutes away."

"OK D-D," Sam says, not looking away from our mom.

It feels so good to breathe the outside air. After four days of hospital food amid the stench of death, I feel a little guilty at my relief to get out of there.

The next morning, I return to the hospital while Jack drives to the airport to pick up Rose. I haven't seen Rose in six weeks and though I feel badly she's coming home to such sadness, I just can't wait to kiss her plump cheeks and hold her soft warm hands.

"I didn't sleep all night," Sam tells me.

"Tell me about it," I tell him, refreshed with nine hours of sleep in me. "Hi Mom. I love you."

I feel like I just can't say those words enough. I want her to hear it over and over.

"I'm outta here," Sam announces. "I have to shower and get something to eat and sleep."

"No, come on," I complain. "You just got here last night."

"I'll be back later," he promises.

"What time?" I badger him.

"I don't know. When I get here," he says.

"OK, well, keep your cell phone on in case something happens. And don't stay away all day!"

Irked at my admonishment, Sam leaves.

Kathy's no longer screaming out in anguish. In fact, she is snoring so loudly you can hear it down the hallway. But it's not really a snore. It's the death rattle.

The door to her room opens again — it's a nurse with a hospitality cart for the family. Loaded with apples and cookies and juice boxes, it's a sweet gesture on behalf of the hospital. The staff only come in the room now to ask if *we* need anything. We've been here four days and they haven't asked us once when we're leaving. While there was talk at one point of taking my mother back to her home, we all decided the trip would probably kill her, and they welcomed us to see out her life in her sun-filled hospital room.

"Hi," says Rose, coming in behind the nurse. At 18 years of age, tan and over six feet tall in her hipster dress, it is like someone from another planet has entered. Though she's only been gone six weeks, she feels years older to me. I rush to hug her and bury my nose in her hair. "Oh, Mama," she says, in part because I have so little hair and I look really "cancery," in part because she knows she's about to reckon with her grandmother's death, and in part because she's home and wrapped in her mother's arms.

"I'm so glad you're here! You look so beautiful," I say, stepping aside. "This is it honey. Nana's been waiting for you. Go to her. Touch her. Let her know you're here. And tell her what you want her to hear from you."

She floats to Kathy's bedside, taking her hand and kissing her forehead.

"Hi Nana, it's me, Rose," she tells her.

I don't know what Rose says. She speaks so quietly, sharing one last intimate moment with a woman who played an integral part in her upbringing. When she finishes, she comes to my side — tears streaking down her face — and sits on the cot that the hospital has placed in the room for the family.

There's a shift in the room. My mother's soul, which feels as if it has been expanding and filling the whole room over the past few days, seems to release. The puzzle is finished. Her closest surviving family has checked in. And Kathy is letting go.

When Sam returns later in the day, I ask if he can stay the night with her again. I can feel that these are the last hours of my mother's life and I want Sam to usher my mother through her death. She and Sam have always had a special bond, and I just feel that my mother wants Sam to be her final companion. Though I would like to be with her as she lets go, I can't explain how I know he needs to be by her side — alone — at that moment.

Just as it is a gift to usher someone into this world, I believe it is a gift to usher them out.

I sit in the room with Kathy as the last train of family and friends filter into the room and say their goodbyes. At around 10 p.m. I stand.

I know when I walk out that door, this will be the last time I see my mother alive.

"OK, Sam," I tell him, taking a deep breath. Rose and Jack and everyone else left hours ago. "I'll be here in the morning."

"'K, D-D," he says.

I turn to my mom. My beautiful silly mom.

"You have been … the best Mom," I say, kissing her cold cheek, sure that this is my last farewell. "Thank you. Thank you. Thank you. I love you … so much. I'll see you in the next world. Goodbye, Mom."

The next morning, Sam calls me as I'm leaving for the hospital.

"She's gone," is all he says.

There are these moments in life where time slows down, sound mutes, and the outside world becomes a blur. For me, they're easy to list: When Jack first told me he loved me; when Rose was born; when my father died; when I was diagnosed with terminal brain cancer; and now, when my mother died. Though I can't remember it, I imagine my birth was muted too, passing from one state into another.

Death — the punctuation that corporeal existence has ended — is the unassailable reminder that our imminent demise is just a paragraph or two away.

After Kathy's body grows cold, Sam, Don, Rose, Ada, Jack and I thank the hospital staff and head back to my house in relative silence. Words seem superfluous at this moment.

I feel rudderless. I feel abandoned. I feel tired. I feel deeply sad. But I also feel relief that Kathy's pain has ended. Diagnosed with Alzheimer's in her 50s, she's been valiantly fighting the disease for almost thirty years. As she struggled to hold onto her relevance and legitimacy, she stood up to the beast that was crushing her and fought like a warrior. She never lost her sense of humor. She never backed down from responsibility to her family or her patients. And she never quit loving. Having grown up in that shadow of her black-belt attitude was the greatest training I could have asked for as I faced my cancer. I knew to stand up, pull out my daggers, and swing. Swing like a motherfucker. Swing for my life.

Yes, I'm still tired. Yes I'm still forgetful. Yes I'm still menopausal. Yes my joints and feet still hurt. And no, I still can't skip. But goddammit, I'm alive. For now, my tumor has been rendered inert. She is still in my head — but she lost this round. And while there is no guarantee that she won't reanimate, I don't care. The medical world has more daggers up its sleeve. And for today — I'm here, with my family and my friends, chasing my dreams, cracking my jokes, and hanging out in my little life until the next muted moment comes along. In the midst of my tears over Kathy's loss, I glow with the joy that I still have the only thing that any of us have.

I have today.

ACKNOWLEDGMENTS

Here's the problem with acknowledgments. No matter how scrupulously you scour the list of everyone who was part of this story, you're going to forget one name, and that person will be so hurt. So here goes, and if you're part of an amalgamation, know that I appreciated every big and small effort you all made.

I would like to start with my doctors, nurses, technicians, Reiki healers, massage therapists and my acupuncturist. Quite simply, you all saved my life. Thank you.

To my cancer buddies at University of Washington and Procure, your camaraderie was priceless. Thank you.

Don, Ada, Kimmie and Jack, your assistance at checkups and meeting doctors and taking me to numerous appointments kept the boat sailing straight in a stormy sea. Thank you.

And a special shoutout to Ada. I can't believe you upended your life and MOVED TO SEATTLE from Albuquerque to help me, not only with my cancer, but with my mom and with the laborious challenge of cleaning out my parents' home and prepping it for sale. Wow, you just went beyond the call of duty! Thank you.

Jim and Libby, you found out my diagnosis with me and you were just so quietly supportive throughout the whole game that I felt A-OK whenever you were around. Thank you.

Al and Sue, you were the first to jump in and prepare me for the battle, with medical advice, relevant reading and overall support. Thank you.

Mia and Susan, you traveled here to hold my hand and rub my aching head and feet. Thank you.

Leslie. What what? You left a funny card on my doorstep EVERY DAY during radiation and many days throughout the rest of treatment. I never properly thanked you, but please know that I came to anticipate the daily gesture with expectant pleasure. Thank you.

Abby, I'd never heard of meal train until you organized one for our family. Being released from the task of shopping and cooking was immeasurably helpful. I sat on the sofa every day with gripping anticipation of 6 o'clock, willing a knock on the door that promised the latest beautiful dinner from my friends (and yours) baring pots and platters of beautifully prepared meals, often from backyard veggie gardens! Thank you.

Kat, Mike, Shafeen, Carrie, Neal and Mary. Really? A professional Vitamix Mixer and weekly deliveries of organic greens for my daily smoothies? I do have to admit, I hated those smoothies, but I also believe they played a part in my healing. Thank you.

Annette darling, thank you for the perfect book cover. And Abby, for formatting the book and letting me take over your computer for days at a time to finish the book! Thanks to both of you.

Alycia, Daniel, Marty, Rachel, Helen, Darryl, Andrea, Monica and Anne, god I value your friendship. Knowing just what to say and how to say it, you helped me avert despair and focus on survival (with plenty of yuks and giggles). Thank you.

Corbin, your helpful editing improved my work, kept me on track, and coached me at a time when I really needed a fire under my ass. Thank you.

Theo, for introducing me to the art of memoir.

Paula, for helping me maintain my dignity and sense of humor. Thank you.

Saul, for being an elegant, gracious, calming presence during this period.

Hadley, Sophie and Augusta, for being there for Rose when I couldn't. Thank you.

And to everyone else who sent prayer cards and blankets and flowers and who called and texted just to say "Hi" and "I love you." Thank you.

Oh, and Arthur. Thank you for staying by Kathy's side as she tried to hold onto her mind. And thank you for being such comforting and devoted company during my treatment. Who's a good boy? You are! Here's a treat! Nooo, you have to sit for it. Good boy! And thank you.

Jack, thank you for making me feel loved throughout the drama.

Rose, thank you for being the love of my life. You and you alone gave me a reason to fight. I love you. Mom

CPSIA information can be obtained
at www.ICGtesting.com
Printed in the USA
LVHW090159280619
622634LV00001B/29/P

9 780991 105052